Understanding and Controlling Stuttering

THE SECOND EDITION

(Third Printing)

Understanding & Controlling Stuttering

A Comprehensive New Approach Based on the Valsalva Hypothesis

by William D. Parry, Esq.

Illustrations by Amie Rumsey

Distributed in Cooperation with the
NATIONAL STUTTERING ASSOCIATION
New York, New York

In memory of my parents,
Mary E. Parry and William B. Parry

Copyright © 2000, 2004 by William D. Parry.
Previous editions copyright © 1992, 1993, 1994 by William D. Parry.
Third Printing (updated) 2004

All rights reserved. Printed in the U. S. A.

No part of this publication may be reproduced or transmitted in any form or by any means without permission in writing from the author.

Published by William D. Parry,
520 Baird Road, Merion Station, PA 19066

Distributed in cooperation with the
National Stuttering Association
119 W. 40th Street, 14th Floor, New York, NY 10018
Telephone: 1-800-WE STUTTER
e-mail: info@WeStutter.org
Website: www.WeStutter.org

Cover design by Bob Lombardo

ISBN 1-929773-01-3

To the Reader:

This book is not intended to take the place of diagnosis and treatment by a qualified medical specialist or speech-language pathologist. Comments may be addressed to:

William D. Parry, 520 Baird Road, Merion Station, PA 19066
Telephone: 215-735-3500 (office); 610-664-5139 (home)
e-mail: **valsalvastutter@aol.com**

Visit the **Valsalva Stuttering Network** website at
www.valsalva.org

Table of Contents

	Preface	vii
	Acknowledgements	x
Part I.	**The Puzzle of Stuttering**	1
Chapter 1.	The Stuttering Experience	2
Chapter 2.	The Stutterer's Quandary	6
Chapter 3.	Pieces of the Puzzle	9
Part II.	**Speech and the Valsalva Mechanism**	13
Chapter 4.	The Speech Mechanism	14
Chapter 5.	The Basics of Speech	19
Chapter 6.	The Valsalva Mechanism	23
Part III.	**The Valsalva Hypothesis**	29
Chapter 7.	An Introduction to the Valsalva Hypothesis	30
Chapter 8.	Valsalva Tuning and the Stuttering Block	34
Chapter 9.	Valsalva Tuning and Phonation	37
Part IV.	**Perpetuation of Stuttering Behavior**	41
Chapter 10.	Varieties of Stuttering	42
Chapter 11.	The Valsalva-Stuttering Cycle	46
Chapter 12.	The Psychology of Stuttering	50
Part V.	**Susceptibility to Stuttering**	55
Chapter 13.	The Origins of Stuttering	56
Chapter 14.	Speech Functions of the Brain	61
Chapter 15.	Heredity and the Stutterer's Brain	65
Chapter 16.	The Brain and the Valsalva Mechanism	72

Part VI.	**Fluency Enhancing Conditions**	77
Chapter 17.	A New Perspective on Fluency Techniques	78
Chapter 18.	The Effects of Hearing and Role Playing	83
Part VII.	**Stuttering Therapy**	89
Chapter 19.	Stuttering Therapies Revisited	90
Chapter 20.	Psychological Approaches to Therapy	97
Chapter 21.	Behavior-Oriented Therapies	102
Chapter 22.	Self-Help for Stuttering	108
Part VIII.	**Breaking the Valsalva-Stuttering Cycle**	113
Chapter 23.	The Principles of Valsalva Control	114
Chapter 24.	Adopting a Valsalva-Free Attitude	119
Chapter 25.	Exercises for Valsalva Control	123
Chapter 26.	Phonation Exercises	128
Chapter 27.	Valsalva Control for Everyday Speech	133
Chapter 28.	Learning from Experience	137
Conclusion.	**A New Outlook on Stuttering**	141
	Appendices	147
Appendix A.	A Voyage to Adronia	149
Appendix B.	Organizations for Stuttering Information and Self-Help	155
	Bibliography	157
	Index	162

Preface

THIS IS THE BOOK I wish I could have read many years ago, back when I started high school as a teenager with a severe stuttering problem. I had stuttered since age four, but adolescence was when the agony really began. Although I started as a straight-A student, winner of the school science fair, and president of the freshman class, my struggle with stuttering soon turned my life into a nightmare of frustration, embarrassment, shame, anger, and even doubts about my own sanity.

Through elocution lessons, I had developed a fine speaking voice and the ability to act out roles in front of audiences with perfect fluency. This convinced me that there was nothing basically wrong with my vocal mechanism. However, in ordinary speech, my stuttering was becoming worse than ever. What could explain this paradox? And what could account for the tendency to stutter more in some situations, or on some words, than others? Was my problem all "psychological"? Was I neurotic or crazy?

Thus began my personal quest to understand and control my stuttering. Over the next three decades I read books on stuttering and psychology, volunteered for experiments and studies, and submitted to a wide range of treatments. These included speech therapy at a number of university clinics, psychological counseling, and many years of intensive psychoanalysis (based on the then-prevalent notion that stuttering was caused by unconscious emotional problems). None of these did very much to resolve my stuttering.

I finally quit psychoanalysis in frustration, because of the analyst's insistence that the cause of stuttering was purely psychological, without any physiological component. However, I did not fare much better with various behavior-type therapies — such as those using the miniature metronome or the "airflow" technique. I hated the monotonous and unnatural sound of these "artificial fluency" methods and found that I soon relapsed back into stuttering. Furthermore, these approaches did not give me a satisfactory understanding of *why* I stuttered, or exactly how the psychological and physical factors interacted to cause stuttering in some instances but not in others.

At the moment of stuttering, it seemed as if a mysterious "switch" was thrown that caused a vise to clamp down on my speech. I suspected that the "switch" was physiological in nature, but that it was tripped by psychological factors. I hoped that, by discovering the exact mechanism involved, I would have a rational basis for understanding and controlling the problem.

After terminating all therapy, I continued to search for the answer through personal experimentation, extensive review of medical literature, and consultations with professional researchers in the fields of laryngology and speech pathology. I studied hundreds of books and articles on not only stuttering, but also related areas of anatomy, neurology, and speech production. I met with researchers at the Temple University Speech Department and the Pennsylvania Hospital Department of Laryngology, and corresponded with other experts around the United States. On one occasion, I had a fiber-optic tube inserted through my nasal passage and down my throat to obtain videotapes of my larynx in action.

Through these efforts, I found what I believe to be the physiological "switch" to my stuttering. It is called the **Valsalva mechanism** — a neurologically coordinated combination of muscles in the larynx, mouth, chest, and abdomen. Its normal function is to assist us in exerting strenuous physical effort or in forcing things out of the body (as in defecation). However, if we mistakenly activate the Valsalva mechanism during our effort to speak, I believe it may cause a forceful blockage of airflow or an interference with phonation — two of the basic, underlying elements of stuttering.

This mechanism perfectly described the symptoms I experienced during stuttering. It explained why stuttering was more likely to occur when I felt the need to "try hard" to speak or to "force out" the words. It was also consistent with nearly all the facts I knew about stuttering, both through my own observations and my reading. However, I could find *nothing* about the Valsalva mechanism in any of the literature on stuttering — except for a few studies in Czechoslovakia that were later brought to my attention.

Spurred on by the thrill of discovery, I proceeded to formulate what I called the "Valsalva Hypothesis." Briefly stated, it shows how stuttering may result from *a neurological confusion between two normal bodily functions* — the voice and the Valsalva mechanism. I first mentioned these ideas in a short article, "Finding My Way Out of the Woods," which appeared in the January 1985 issue of the National Stuttering Project's newsletter, *Letting Go*. A longer paper, "Stuttering and the Valsalva Mechanism: A Hypothesis in Need of Investigation," was subsequently published in the December 1985 issue of *The Journal of Fluency Disorders*.

Although the Valsalva Hypothesis has not been tested scientifically, and therefore has been neither proved nor disproved, it provides a "working hypothesis" which explains the complexities of stuttering better than any other theory I have seen.

The more I worked on my hypothesis, the more the contradictions and paradoxes of stuttering made sense. After a lifetime of frustration and confusion, the pieces of the puzzle were finally falling into place. Through these insights I was, for the first time, able to get a "handle" on my problem. I was able to develop exercises and approaches to speech that increased my fluency dramatically. My speech improved to such a degree that I was soon able to function comfortably in the highly stressful and speech-intensive position of a *trial lawyer* — a goal that I had dreamed of for many years.

Having found the Valsalva Hypothesis to be of great value in my own case, I was eager to learn whether it might be helpful to other persons who stuttered. My desire to share and test these ideas led me to the National Stuttering Project (now known as the National Stuttering Association), a non-profit self-help organization. With the help and encouragement of its Executive Director, John Ahlbach, I founded the Philadelphia Area Chapter of the NSP in January 1985. I led the chapter and facilitated its self-help/support meetings for the next 15 years. In 1996, I was elected to the NSP's Board of Directors and became Chair of its Advocacy Committee.

It was also my pleasure to work with Robert Gathman, the president and founder of Speak Easy International Foundation, Inc., headquartered in New Jersey.

Over the years, I have met hundreds of people who stutter — not only at our local chapter meetings, but also at workshops and conventions of the NSP/NSA, Speak Easy International, the Canadian Association for People Who Stutter, and international conventions for people who stutter. I have given numerous workshops and presentations about the Valsalva Hypothesis at these gatherings, and the positive responses have strengthened my conviction that this approach is worthy of serious pursuit.

In August 1992, I presented two workshops on the Valsalva Hypothesis at the Third International Convention of People Who Stutter, held in San Francisco, where I also introduced a special preliminary edition of this book. The first completed edition of this book was published in 1994.

In 1995, I was invited to give a major presentation and workshop at the World Congress for People Who Stutter, held in Linköping, Sweden. I subsequently adapted my Sweden speech into an article, "The Valsalva Mechanism: A Key to Understanding and Controlling Stuttering," which I published on the Internet. That article has elicited enthusiastic e-mail from hundreds of stutterers all over the world — many declaring that the Valsalva

Hypothesis described their stuttering experience more precisely than anything they had ever encountered.

This has been the first book to deal with stuttering in terms of the Valsalva Hypothesis. It is intended primarily for the adult or adolescent person who stutters, but hopefully it will also be of interest to therapists and others concerned with the problem. It does not offer any quick and easy gimmicks to "cure" stuttering. Instead, its approach requires that we first gain a thorough *understanding* of what stuttering is and why we do it. Only then are we ready to master the principles of *controlling* stuttering.

Based on insights gained from the Valsalva Hypothesis, this book will present a comprehensive view of stuttering, including both its physical and psychological aspects. It will show how these factors may interact to cause and perpetuate stuttering through the "Valsalva-Stuttering Cycle." In this way, we shall attempt to explain virtually every aspect of stuttering behavior, its paradoxes, its causes, and its treatment. We shall analyze the symptoms and circumstances of stuttering, the development of stuttering in childhood, the influence of heredity and neurological factors, and the physical and psychological conditions that tend to increase or reduce stuttering.

These discussions have been organized with the lay reader in mind, starting out as simply as possible and then gradually introducing more and more complexity as we go along. To ease the way, I have tried to avoid scientific jargon and to explain the physiological aspects of speech in simple, everyday terms. Likewise, I have chosen to use the ordinary English alphabet — instead of the scientifically preferred phonetic alphabet — in representing the various sounds of speech. (I hope that professional speech-language pathologists will not find this too disconcerting.)

We shall then proceed to discuss the strengths and weaknesses of existing therapies, point out the elements that many of them have in common, show why most stutterers tend to relapse, and indicate ways in which therapies might be made more effective. Finally, we shall suggest an experimental program of self-therapy that incorporates both physical and psychological techniques aimed at controlling the Valsalva mechanism and breaking the stuttering cycle.

Of course, there is no guaranty that any method will bring fluency to everyone. It would be extremely presumptuous to claim that anyone will be "cured" of stuttering just by reading a book. However, if this book helps even *one* person to get a better handle on his or her stuttering, it will have served its purpose.

Acknowledgements

I am indebted to the many people who have contributed to my understanding of stuttering: researchers around the world who have provided a growing foundation of scientific data; speech-language pathologists who have given advice and sent me articles and information; and members of the stuttering self-help movement who have shared their personal insights and experiences. While there was often disagreement on many points, the sharing of diverse views about stuttering helped me continually to refine and strengthen my ideas.

Special thanks go to C. Woodruff Starkweather, Ph.D., for his consultations and review of my original paper on "Stuttering and the Valsalva Mechanism"; to the *Journal of Fluency Disorders* for publishing it; to Joseph P. Atkins, Jr., M.D., of the Pennsylvania Hospital Department of Otolaryngology, who performed a fiber-optic study of my larynx and who also reviewed that paper prior to publication; and to Keith Young, Ph.D., for his practical advice on presenting my hypothesis.

Others who have been valuable resources include John Paul Brady, M.D., of the University of Pennsylvania Department of Psychiatry; speech therapist Burnetta Swartz; and numerous other therapists and speech-language pathologists whom I have met through our local chapter of the National Stuttering Project. I also appreciate the comments and suggestions I have received in response to the preliminary edition of this book, including those from Arnold H. Gessel, M.D.; Professor Don Mowrer of Arizona State University;

Dr. E. Vervaet of the Netherlands; Herbert G. Goldberg, of the Foundation for Fluency, Inc.; Dr. Eugene B. Cooper of the University of Alabama Speech and Hearing Center; Jock Carlisle; Melvin Powers; and many others.

Particularly crucial to this endeavor was the help I have received from members of the stuttering self-help movement. First and foremost, I wish to credit John Harrison, Program Director of the National Stuttering Association (formerly the National Stuttering Project), who gave me the encouragement and moral support to complete this book, and who did more than anyone to bring the Valsalva Hypothesis to the attention of stutterers and researchers around the world.

Thanks also to Dr. E. Robert "Cy" Libby, Dan Weiss, Agnes McGerty, and other members of the Philadelphia Area Chapter of the NSP; to John Ahlbach, former Executive Director of the NSP; Robert Gathman, President of Speak Easy Int'l Foundation, Inc.; Mike Hughes, Executive Director of Speak Easy, Inc. (Canada); Rodney Gabel; and to everyone who has participated in my Valsalva workshops. Thanks also to the National Stuttering Association's current Executive Director, Annie Bradberry, and to Tammy Flores at the NSA office.

Finally, my deepest appreciation is reserved for my wife Andrea and my daughters, Sara and Jessica, for their help, cooperation, and support during the long hours while I was engrossed in this project.

Part I.

The Puzzle of Stuttering

CHAPTER 1.

The Stuttering Experience

WE LIVE IN A WORLD dominated by the spoken word. Almost everywhere — at home, school, work, social gatherings — speech is the way people get to know one another and share ideas, information, and feelings. By means of speech, we tell who we are, what we want, and why we are important. Through the give and take of spoken conversation, we develop friendships and become skilled in dealing with others. Speech is like a magic thread by which we weave ourselves into the fabric of society.

It is easy for the average person to take speech for granted. When an idea springs into his mind, he simply opens his mouth. Automatically, his brain comes up with the right words and sends them off through the organs of speech. Almost instantly — without any conscious effort — he hears himself talking. He gives no thought to the complex interaction of brain cells, nerves, muscles, and other parts of the body that make his speech possible. The words just seem to flow, like the clear water of a mountain stream.

To be sure, the average person may find some speaking situations more difficult. Answering a question in class, asking the boss for a raise, delivering a speech to a large audience, for example. The person may be unsure of what to say, afraid of angering someone, or worried about making a fool of himself. Rarely, however, will he doubt his ability to speak. Frightened and hesitant though he may be, he will nevertheless open his mouth, and the magic of speech will take over.

But this is not true for the person who stutters.

For the person who stutters, speaking is an entirely different experience. Speech doesn't flow smoothly, like the babbling mountain brook. Speech is more like the poor salmon, struggling to jump over waterfalls as it fights its way upstream to the spawning ground.

If you are a stutterer, you have no assurance that the words will spring from your lips on command. True, there are times when your speech may come easily. But in other situations, the flow of speech is blocked.

Sometimes, when you try to say a word, your speech is so totally blocked that nothing comes out at all. The blocking may occur in the mouth, with your lips or teeth pressing tightly together like a vise. Or your tongue may feel like it's trying to push its way through the roof of your mouth. Sometimes the air gets strangled down in your throat, and you feel as if you had swallowed a cork. Other times your vocal cords seem frozen, unable to make a sound. You may grope desperately for words, but all you get are *uh*'s and *ah*'s and other embarrassing noises.

Sometimes the block is partial or intermittent. You may get stuck on a certain sound and keep prolonging it. For example, your pronunciation of "s-s-s-s-s-s-s-snake" may hiss like the serpent it describes. Or you may keep repeating the first part of a word over and over, before being able to move onto the rest. When you say "buh-buh-buh-buh-basketball," you may give the impression that you're actually dribbling the ball down the court.

But stuttering is not simply the repetition of sounds we see in the written depictions of stuttered speech. The hallmark of real stuttering is the tremendous amount of *physical effort* a stutterer uses in trying to force out the words. Instead of touching lightly and briefly during speech, the lips and tongue press harder and longer than necessary, or the larynx itself may clamp shut. While this is happening, the air pressure in the stutterer's body may increase to the point that he feels he is about to explode.

In addition to the blocks, stuttering is often complicated by other kinds of physical and verbal behavior. In the struggle to force the words out, a stutterer might twist and contort his face, jerk his head, blink his eyes, grind his teeth, bite the inside of his mouth, swing his arms, etc. He may insert unnecessary words, phrases, or sounds as "starters" before trying to say a difficult word. He may go back and repeat the previous few words over and over and over, as he tries again and again to leap over the hurdle. If possible, he may try to substitute a different word that is easier to say.

Persons who stutter are generally able to sense that a particular word is going to be trouble, even before they try to say it. Therefore, some stutterers become adept at **covert stuttering** — struggling silently through the blocks before speaking, changing and censoring words in advance, and saying only the things they feel will not give them trouble. Their entire conversation is dictated by the effort to conceal their stuttering. Other stutterers go to equally great lengths to avoid talking altogether.

The Definition of Stuttering

The precise definition of "stuttering" is a matter on which speech pathologists often disagree. Therefore, it may be helpful to explain exactly what is meant by the term when used in this book.

Stuttering refers to a particular speech disorder in which the flow of speech tends to be involuntarily disrupted by forceful closures of the mouth or larynx, by repetitions or prolongations of sounds and syllables, or by hesitations or delays in making voiced sounds. Stuttering generally involves an excessive amount of effort, force, and struggle in the attempt to speak. It also may be accompanied by a variety of behaviors intended to avoid, postpone, or hide the blocks.

Stuttering is sometimes called "stammering," especially in Great Britain. For our purposes, the two words are synonymous and both refer to the same disorder.

Stuttering must be distinguished from **disfluency**, which refers broadly to any interruption in the natural flow and rhythm of speech. Stuttering is a very specific *kind* of disfluency. Many people are disfluent from time to time, for a variety of reasons, but that doesn't necessarily make them stutterers. Stuttering also differs from language disabilities such as **aphasia**, in which the ability to think of the appropriate words is impaired. A stutterer's problem is not in *finding* the words, but rather in *saying* them.

We must also differentiate stuttering from a relatively rare kind of disfluency, sometimes called **acquired stuttering**, which may occur at any age following certain kinds of brain damage. Although it may involve stuttering-like symptoms, acquired stuttering is actually a very different disorder, as will be explained in a subsequent chapter. This book will be devoted exclusively to the usual, garden variety of stuttering — sometimes called **developmental stuttering** — which seems to develop of its own accord during childhood. Therefore, the discussions in this book may have little or no application to a brain-damaged person with acquired stuttering.

Developmental stutterers, as distinguished from acquired stutterers, are generally capable of fluent speech in at least some instances. Most have no trouble when singing or when reading in unison with someone else, and they are usually much more fluent when talking to themselves or to animals or small children. The severity of developmental stuttering often depends on the speaking situation. For example, many individuals have a particularly hard time saying their name, talking on the telephone, or addressing authority figures.

Those are some of the basic characteristics of stuttering. The severity, frequency, and situations in which stuttering occurs will vary according to each individual. We will examine all of these aspects of stuttering in greater detail as we go along.

The Prevalence of Stuttering

If you stutter, you have probably experienced the feeling of being alone and out of place in our glib and garrulous world. But you are not the only one. It has been estimated that nearly one percent of the general population stutters. This would amount to more than two million stutterers in the United States alone. For some reason, stuttering is about four times more common in males than females.

There is truth to the statement, "If you stutter you are in good company." Throughout history, there have been many notable people who stuttered. These include Moses, Aristotle, Virgil, Sir Isaac Newton, Joseph Priestley, Charles Darwin, Lewis Carroll, Charles Lamb, Clara Barton, Sir Winston Churchill, King George VI of England, W. Somerset Maugham, James Earl Jones, and many others.

Stuttering usually starts in childhood, most often between ages two and eight (although in rare cases it may begin much later). Roughly 4 to 5 per cent of people experience stuttering at some time during their childhood. Fortunately, the majority become fluent by the time they reach adulthood, even without speech therapy. But the rest are not so lucky. Many go on to become adult stutterers, for whom stuttering is likely to be a chronic, persistent problem for the rest of their lives.

The Impact of Stuttering

If you stutter, you know that the experience of stuttering is far more than just the blocks themselves. It can affect one's entire life.

The experience of stuttering is the constant fear of speaking situations, the fear of ridicule and rejection. It is the uncertainty of not knowing whether the words will come out when you need them, or whether you will suddenly find yourself abandoned by speech in an awkward situation. It is the frustration of not being able to say what you want, of having important words bottled up inside you while other people babble nonsense with no trouble at all.

Stuttering is the embarrassment of not being able to say your name when meeting someone. It is the exhausting struggle to tell people even the most routine information, such as your address and telephone number. It is the isolation of not being able to participate fully in everyday conversations.

Stuttering is the inconvenience of walking or driving from store to store in search of an item, because you can't use the telephone to call ahead to see who has it. It is the disappointment of not being able to order the food you want in a restaurant, and selecting an alternative that is easier to say.

Stuttering is the disillusionment of seeing a job or promotion go to a less qualified but more fluent person. It is the resignation of settling for a job or career that is less rewarding than the one you really wanted, simply because it doesn't require you to talk as much.

The experience of stuttering is the pervasive feeling of shame and guilt, and nagging doubts about your competence and worthiness as a person. It is the sense of forever being a little child, while other people are self-confident adults.

And it is the indignity of constantly having to put up with people who tell you to "relax," who try to fill in words for you, or who keep giving you useless advice on how to stop stuttering.

General References

ANDREWS, G., CRAIG, A., FEYER, A., HODDINOTT, S., HOWIE, P., & NEILSON, M. Stuttering: a review of research findings and theories circa 1982. *Journal of Speech and Hearing Disorders,* 1983, 48, 226-246.
BLOODSTEIN, O. *A Handbook on Stuttering.* 5th ed. San Diego: Singular Publishing Group, 1995.
BLOODSTEIN, O. *Stuttering: The Search for a Cause and Cure.* Needham Heights, MA: Allyn & Bacon, 1993.
BOBRICK, B. *Knotted Tongues.* New York: Simon & Schuster, 1995.
CARLISLE, J. A. *Tangled Tongue.* Reading, MA: Addison-Wesley Publishing Co., 1985.
COOPER, E. B. *Understanding Stuttering: Information for Parents.* Chicago: National Easter Seal Society, 1990.
JEZER, M. *Stuttering: A Life Bound Up in Words.* New York: Basic Books, 1997.
KEHOE, T. D. *Stuttering: Science, Therapy & Practice.* Boulder, CO: Casa Futura Technologies, 1999.
MURRAY, F. P. *A Stutterer's Story.* Memphis, TN: Stuttering Foundation of America, 1991.
ROSENFIELD, D. B. Stuttering. *Current Problems in Pediatrics,* 1982, 12, No. 8.
SHAMES, G. H., AND RUBIN, H., EDITORS. *Stuttering Then and Now.* Columbus, OH: Charles E. Merrill Publishing

STARKWEATHER, C. W. *Fluency and Stuttering.* Englewood Cliffs, N.J.: Prentice-Hall, 1987.
STARKWEATHER, C. W., & GIVENS-ACKERMAN, J. *Stuttering.* Austin, TX: Pro-Ed, 1997.
VAN RIPER, C. *The Nature of Stuttering.* 2nd ed. Englewood Cliffs, N.J.: Prentice-Hall, 1982.
WINGATE, M. E. *Stuttering: Theory and Treatment.* New York: Irvington, 1976.

CHAPTER 2.

The Stutterer's Quandary

ONCE THERE WAS a student who stuttered very badly. Whenever he had to stand in front of the class to give an oral report, he couldn't say anything, no matter how hard he tried. All that came out was, "Uh-uh-uh-uh... Uh-uh-uh-uh..."

The teacher was a great believer in the power of positive thinking. One day he took the student aside.

"Listen. I know how you can overcome your stuttering. All you need is self-confidence. From now on, I want you to stand up straight, look people in the eye, and keep telling yourself, 'I can say it! I can say it!'"

The student took this advice to heart. A week later, he was called on to deliver another oral report. This time, he strode confidently to the front of the room, stood up straight, looked his classmates in the eye, and began:

"Uh-uh-uh-uh... I can say it! I can say it! Uh-uh-uh-uh... I can say it! I can say it!"

The preceding story illustrates a recurring experience — well-intentioned, simplistic advice that fails because it doesn't get to the heart of the problem. I myself have tried the same approach as in the story, with similar results. For years I used the slogan, "I can say it," as a crutch, silently mouthing those words over and over when I came to a block. It didn't help one bit. Instead, it became just another part of my stuttering behavior.

Stuttering, while not the worst of handicaps, certainly can be one of the most frustrating. As bad as other handicaps may be, at least they are consistent. Everybody accepts the fact that disabilities like blindness and paralysis have physical causes beyond the victim's control. The disability is always there, and the handicapped person and those around him must learn to accept and adapt to it. No one keeps insisting that the person would be cured if only he would "think positive" or "relax."

Stuttering is different. Although everybody is quick to voice an opinion, no one really knows for sure what causes it or how it can be cured. Despite recent experiments to discover the effects of various drugs on stuttering, medical science has yet to find a "pink pill" that will make the problem disappear.

Unlike other disabilities, stuttering has the mystifying and maddening habit of coming and going. Even if you stutter badly, chances are that you will be perfectly fluent when singing, talking in unison with other people, and in certain speaking situations. You may do a great job acting out a role on stage, but not be able to say your name when asked. You may begin telling a joke with perfect fluency, but not be able to deliver the punch line. You may have long stretches of fluency when it really doesn't matter. Then, just when the words are most important, stuttering jumps out of the closet and pins your speech to the ground.

People find these paradoxes difficult to understand. If you can speak normally *some* of the time, they may ask, what excuse do you have for not speaking normally *all* of the time? Instead of appreciating the seriousness of your predicament, some people may see your stuttering as an object of ridicule. Even worse, they may suspect that you are mentally defective or emotionally disturbed. Before long, you may start wondering the same things yourself. The worst torments are probably those inflicted by stutterers upon themselves — including feelings of shame, guilt, personal failure, low self-esteem, and even doubts about their own sanity.

While modern scientists have made important discoveries about stuttering, they have yet to produce definite answers about its cause and cure. Controversies continue to rage over whether stuttering is caused by emotional problems, learned behavior, heredity, or possible defects in the brain or nervous system. Reading through the enormous array of books and articles on the subject, one gets the impression that *almost nothing* can be said about stuttering that will not be contradicted by other experts with a different viewpoint. Persons who stutter are also confronted with conflicting claims about a wide variety of competing treatment methods. These range from psychotherapy to various forms of behavior modification, "fluency shaping" programs, drugs, and electronic devices to be worn while speaking. It is difficult for the stutterer to know *what* to believe.

Psychological Views of Stuttering

For many years, stuttering was viewed by the experts as being primarily a *psychological* or *emotional* disorder. The root of the problem was thought to be some deep, emotional conflict, locked away in the unconscious mind. Stutterers were prescribed various forms of psychotherapy. They discussed their feelings, analyzed their dreams, dredged up childhood memories, and complained about their parents. I myself was shunted down this track. I consulted a string of psychiatrists, read books by Sigmund Freud, and spent more than a decade on an analyst's couch. I dug deeper and deeper into my unconscious mind, searching in vain for the key to my problem. When I *still* kept on stuttering, I figured that I must be even crazier than I had thought!

Other experts dispute the idea that stuttering is an emotional disorder. They point to studies showing that stutterers, as a group, are no more neurotic or emotionally disturbed than the general population, and that psychotherapy, by itself, has not been very successful in treating stuttering. Nevertheless, psychotherapy may be helpful when used in conjunction with other therapies and in dealing with anxieties or emotional problems that a person may have developed as a *result* of the stuttering.

Some experts believe that stuttering is a *learned behavior*. According to one theory, stuttering develops when a child's parents become overly concerned about ordinary childhood disfluency (which most children grow out of) and label it as "stuttering." As a result, the child becomes increasingly anxious about speaking and tries harder and harder not to stutter. This only makes the stuttering worse. According to one expert (Wendell Johnson), "Stuttering is what you do when you try not to stutter."

A part of the "unlearning" process may involve *desensitization*. In the hope of reducing the stutterer's fear of stuttering, he may be instructed to go out and stutter *on purpose*. He may also be taught various techniques of coping with his blocks when they occur.

Neurological Views of Stuttering

Still other experts believe that stuttering is caused by *neurological factors* — such as inherited abnormalities in the brain or nervous system. In support of this theory, they point to studies showing that stuttering often runs in families and that the risk is even greater if you have an identical twin who stutters. In addition, laboratory experiments have shown that stutterers, as a group, are slower than non-stutterers in their reaction times and have slightly different patterns of brain activity. Hardly a year goes by without researchers claiming to have found stutterers to be neurologically abnormal in yet another way. However, the experts disagree as to precisely *what* the crucial defect is and *how* it results in stuttering.

While the neurological theories may help to free stuttering from the stigma of "emotional illness," they have the equally depressing potential of portraying stutterers as being biologically inferior to other people or hopelessly brain-defective. Furthermore, the significance of the research is often blown out of proportion, creating the false impression that the particular trait being studied is the ultimate cause of stuttering. Consequently, we are left with an array of conflicting theories, each attempting to explain some isolated fact, while ignoring other aspects of the stuttering experience. It is no wonder that stutterers feel confused.

Therefore, we must view the research reports cautiously and try to put them in the proper perspective. Even if the tests are accurate, they do not necessarily prove that stuttering is caused by any of the alleged abnormalities. It is possible that some *other* underlying factor might be causing both stuttering and the differences noted.

Although it is possible that certain inherited traits might make some people more *susceptible* to stuttering than others, it is not likely that these are the only factors that determine whether a person is actually going to stutter. Inherited factors alone would not explain why a person stutters *some* of the time but can be fluent at other times. Nor would they explain the cases in which one identical twin stutters but the other twin (with the same genetic material) does not. Or the fact that some stutterers can go on to become totally fluent.

Behavior Modification

Since the 1960's, there has been increasing emphasis on treating stuttering through *behavior modification* — various forms of therapy aimed at changing the *symptoms* of stuttering, rather than looking for underlying causes.

Many of these therapies seek to eliminate the blocks by training the stutterer to use a new method of speaking. This is the "fluency shaping" approach. Depending on the therapy, the stutterer may be taught to slow down his speech, to breathe in a particular way, to ease into the sounds, and to stretch out his words. After a few days, there is a good chance that even the most severe stutterer will be talking fluently. But achieving fluency in the therapist's office is only the first step.

The first big challenge is to carry the fluency out of the clinic and into the real world. For some reason, stutterers have a tremendous resistance to using a new speaking method in everyday situations. Often they complain that it sounds funny or feels unnatural. Once that hurdle is overcome, the next and greatest challenge is to maintain the new-found fluency for more than a few weeks. The rate of relapse is extremely high.

I know this from personal experience. I once received therapy using one of the more publicized methods of instant fluency. I practiced the method diligently, both in the therapist's office and out. After a short time, I had mastered the method and was quite fluent. Even if it did sound a little strange at first, it sure beat stuttering.

But then, after about a month, I could feel the tension and fear starting to creep up on me. Hey, what was this, I wondered? I had thought I was cured. Why was I feeling this way again? I had been told that, as long as I used the method properly, it would be physically *impossible* for me to stutter. Now I wasn't so sure.

One day I unexpectedly bumped into someone I had known before being "cured." As I began to talk, the old fears came crashing down on me. I tried in vain to use the method, but it was too late. I was choked up with stuttering.

Back I was in the Dark Ages. Why?

It didn't matter that I knew the method. It didn't matter that I had conscientiously tried to use it. Suddenly, all my skills and resolve were blown away by the Dark Dragon of Stuttering. The Dark Dragon had just been relaxing in his den for a while, chuckling at my flimsy new armor. Now he had stormed from his cave, and in one breath, had re-established who was boss.

The method had been my little Talisman — a magical charm to protect me from the Dragon of Stuttering. As long as stuttering stayed away, the charm seemed to keep its magic, and I continued to talk. But once stuttering came back, the magic spell was broken. It was impossible to resume using the method with the same confidence as before.

Since I had never been given an accurate understanding as to what really caused stuttering and why the method was supposed to work, I was never able to view it as anything more than a magical trick to give me confidence in speaking. When it failed, the only thing I learned was: *It doesn't work when I really need it!* With my faith shattered, the method seemed worthless.

Some therapists have a tendency to pooh-pooh the stutterer's complaints of failure. They insist that their method works. Instead, they blame the stutterer for failing to use the method properly.

This attitude ignores the most important point: The reason that the stutterer is unable to use a particular speaking method in times of stress may be *the same reason that he stutters in the first place.* Until that reason is understood, the stutterer will continue to be at its mercy, regardless of what speaking method he tries to hide behind.

CHAPTER 3.

Pieces of the Puzzle

HAVE YOU EVER tried to put together one of those giant picture puzzles, made up of a thousand tiny pieces? You open the box, which shows on its lid the beautiful picture you are supposed to make, and find to your dismay a hopeless jumble of cardboard pieces, a total mishmash of colors and shapes. At first, it seems impossible that you could ever put them in order. If you just reached into the pile and tried to fit the pieces together at random, you would soon give up in frustration.

Successfully completing a puzzle requires that we start as simply as possible. First, we must spread out the pieces on the table. Then we find the four corner pieces and the straight-edged pieces that go along the top, bottom, and sides. We concentrate on putting these pieces together first. Once we have the corners and edges linked up, we will have established the outline of the picture. Assembling the rest of the puzzle will now be a lot easier.

Putting together the puzzle of stuttering is a bit more difficult. For one thing, we don't have a picture on the cover of a box to guide us. For another, the corners and edges are not clearly defined. Even worse, we don't know how many of the pieces are missing. Perhaps our picture won't be complete. Nevertheless, we're bound to learn a great deal by doing the best we can with what we've got.

We begin by spreading the pieces on the table — all the facts we know about stuttering, either from our own experience or from scientific studies. Sooner or later we will try to fit *all* of these pieces together, but for the moment we must select a few of them to start with. We are looking first for the corner pieces — the facts that are most fundamental to the stuttering experience.

Circumstances of Stuttering

For the *first* corner piece, let's look for a basic fact that tells about the *kind of circumstances in which we stutter most often or most severely*.

We know that most people who stutter are capable of perfect fluency at certain times. We tend to be more fluent when talking to ourselves, to animals or small children, or to people with whom we feel comfortable.[1] When I was young, I would converse with myself quite fluently as I walked home from school. Sometimes I would go off into the woods and give long, eloquent speeches to the tree stumps.

Stuttering generally increases when we are speaking to authority figures, such as parents, teachers, bosses, policemen, judges, or other people we feel we have to please or impress.[2] It can become particularly bad when the listener seems impatient with our speech and wants us to hurry up. Things become even worse when we are put on the spot in front of a group, with every one waiting for us to get the words out. Imagine standing at a ticket window, with a long line of angry people behind you, as you try to buy a ticket for a train that's just about to pull out of the station. Some stutterers would sooner throw themselves in front of a locomotive than submit to that kind of ordeal.

When we encounter a speaking situation that has given us trouble in the past, stuttering is likely to give a repeat performance. The more we fear that we are going to stutter, the more we usually do. Each individual may have different circumstances that are particularly difficult. Many stutterers (but not all) have an excruciating time whenever they use the telephone. One of my worst phobias was gas stations. I used to drive around with my tank almost empty, because I dreaded asking the gas station attendants to "fill it up." (The arrival of self-service gasoline pumps was a boon to more than one stutterer I know.)

Stuttering is more likely to occur on the most important, precise, or meaningful words in a sentence.[3] When certain words must be said exactly right, like the punch line of a joke, stuttering usually hits the hardest. A prime example is saying your own name — perhaps the biggest bugaboo of every one who stutters. I once heard a story about a man who blocked so severely on his name that he finally changed it to something he could say easily. When the change became legal, he no longer had any trouble with the *old* name, but began blocking like crazy on his *new* name.[4]

In my own experience, I always found it easier to say the *wrong* word, whatever it was, than the precise word that was most appropriate. In answering the telephone, I could not simply say "Hello." In order to get it out, I would have to say "*Yes,* hello." But whenever "yes" was the right word instead of "hello," the situation would be exactly reversed. For example, when the person on the other end immediately said, "Hello, is this Bill Parry?" — I would not be able to say "yes." Now I would have to say, "*Hello,* yes, this is Bill Parry."

One has relative ease in saying words that are unimportant or repetitious. When it is no longer important to say something (for example, after it has been said already), I have heard stutterers (including myself) repeat the same thing over and over again with great fluency.

Is there an underlying fact we can draw from these speaking situations? It seems apparent that stuttering increases when a person is under some kind of "stress." However, this fact alone is a bit too general to serve our purpose. If we look more closely, we will see that all of the above examples involve circumstances in which we feel that the words themselves are especially important, or we anticipate that speaking will be difficult. These are precisely the moments when we are preparing to have trouble talking, when we may feel that some kind of *extra effort* will be needed to get us over the hurdles.

Therefore, I propose that we choose the following basic fact as our first corner piece: *We tend to stutter more when we feel the need to "try hard" and to use extra effort in speaking.*

Symptoms of Stuttering

In the *second* corner of our puzzle, we should probably insert a basic fact that describes the *symptoms of stuttering*. As we look over the pieces, we may be confused, at first, by all the different varieties of stuttering behavior. For example, there are blocks, hesitations, repetitions, prolongations, word substitutions, muscle spasms, gasping for breath, teeth gnashing, avoidance tactics, etc. All of these will eventually have to fit in somewhere. However, it is likely that some of these symptoms are not basic to stuttering, but are merely secondary habits that we have developed in our attempt to *avoid* stuttering.

In selecting our corner piece, let's go directly to the most extreme form of stuttering we know — the total, full-blown stuttering block. You may be painfully familiar with the experience.

You are about to say a word. Your lips or tongue move into the proper position for the first sound. But instead of making a light, momentary contact and then relaxing as they should, they continue to press harder and harder, totally blocking your airflow and preventing any sound from escaping. The harder you try to force the words out, the harder your mouth clamps shut.

When you are trying to say consonants like *b* or *p,* the tight closure is done by the lips. With other consonants, like *d* or *t,* the tongue is involved. If the word starts with a vowel, like *apple,* the forceful closure may occur in the larynx, or voice box, shutting off the airway in the throat.

While the mouth or larynx are clamped shut, the abdominal and chest muscles may tighten up, so as to build up air pressure in the lungs, as if straining to force air through the closure. But the harder we try, the stronger the block becomes.

Of course, there are many instances in which the block is far less severe. Sometimes it is spread out more gradually, through repetitions or prolongations of sounds. But even in these cases, the stutterer is using much more effort and force than normal speech requires.

These observations bring us to our second basic fact: *Stuttering is often characterized by excessive force and effort in the attempt to speak.*[5]

Having established the first two corners of our puzzle, an interesting connection becomes apparent. Both the *circumstances* and the *symptoms* of stuttering seem to be related to *the exertion of effort*. This brings to mind certain remarks of the late Henry Freund, a famous psychiatrist who was once himself a stutterer. He wrote that one of the primary experiences of stuttering is that of "an obstacle which needs force to overcome it,"[6] and that such effort by the stutterer "only increases the force of the closure."[7] Paradoxically, our effort to overcome the "obstacle" to speech becomes the very stuttering behavior that we are trying so hard to avoid.

I myself wrestled with this paradox for most of my life. For example, I knew that when I wanted my car to go forward, I should step on the gas — not stomp on the brakes. Why, then, did I continue to close my mouth tighter and tighter when I tried to speak? No matter how I tried intellectually to recognize the futility of such effort, I found myself at a loss to control it.

At the moment of stuttering, it seemed as if a mysterious "switch" was thrown that caused a vise to clamp down on my speech. I suspected that the "switch" must be physical in nature, but that it might be triggered by psychological factors. This would suggest that we need to find some physical mechanism which would be activated when we feel the need to "try hard," and which would result in the kind of forceful closures that we experience.

Phonation and Stuttering

In addition to forceful closures, there is another symptom that seems basic to much stuttering behavior. This is the difficulty stutterers often have with **phonation** — the vibration of the vocal cords in the larynx that makes the sound of our voice.

Difficulty in phonation is an important factor that most people tend to overlook. For example, most people would say that a stutterer struggling over the word "puh-puh-puh-potato" has trouble pronouncing the *p* sound. But that is obviously not true, since he is saying the *p* perfectly well. His real problem may be in moving on to the *vowel* sound that follows it. There is a delay or inability of his vocal folds in producing the phonation needed to continue the word. When a stutterer makes no attempt to phonate, but simply mouths his words silently — letting people "read his lips" — there is no problem.[8]

Over the past few decades, many speech researchers have found that stutterers have delays in phonation, compared to normal speakers.[9] Several types of stuttering therapy employ various means of teaching improved phonation as a way to increase fluency. When the stutterer learns to concentrate on phonation and vowel sounds, he tends to be more fluent.[10] It should be noted that most stutterers are perfectly fluent when singing — possibly because they must use continuous phonation to carry the melody.[11]

Consequently, we now have a third corner piece: *Stuttering is often characterized by difficulty or delay in phonation.*

This fact gives us an important clue about the physical mechanism that we are seeking. We are looking for a mechanism that would not only encourage forceful closures, but would also inhibit phonation. Since phonation takes place in the larynx, we are looking for a mechanism that would have some effect on that part of the body.

I believe I have found a physical mechanism that meets all these requirements. It is known as the **Valsalva mechanism**. It is a normal bodily function, found in every healthy human being, which is designed to assist us in many types of physical effort. However, if a person activates this mechanism while "trying hard" to speak, it could cause both forceful closures and interference with phonation, leading to stuttering.

Although only one part of the total picture, the Valsalva mechanism is an important key to putting together the many other pieces of the puzzle, which otherwise seem so confusing and contradictory. As we will see in later chapters, the Valsalva mechanism provides an answer to some of the most perplexing paradoxes of stuttering. It explains why certain speech methods tend to promote fluency, and also suggests ways to make therapy more effective.

Before we can fully comprehend how the Valsalva mechanism may be involved in stuttering, we must first get a basic understanding of the physical mechanics of *normal* speech. It's easy to assume that we know how speech works, but have we ever really looked into it? In order to understand what goes wrong, we must know what is *supposed* to happen when everything goes right.

Notes

See Bibliography for complete citations of references.

1. Bloodstein, 1995, p. 297.
2. Bloodstein, 1995, p. 301; Van Riper, 1982, p. 148.
3. Bloodstein, 1995, p. 296; Van Riper, 1982, pp. 151-152.
4. Schwartz, 1976, p. 51.
5. Starkweather, 1987, pp. 37-44; Freund, 1966, pp. 91-100.
6. Freund, 1966, pp. 94-95.
7. Freund, 1966, p. 91.
8. Perkins, Rudas, Johnson, and Bell, 1976.
9. See, e.g., Adams and Reis, 1971; Adams, 1974; Bakker and Brutten, 1989, 1990; Borden, Baer, and Kenney, 1985; Healey and Gutkin, 1984; Mallard, Hicks, and Riggs, 1982; Reich, Till, and Goldsmith, 1981; Starkweather, Hirschman and Tannenbaum, 1976; Starkweather, Franklin, and Smigo, 1984; Starkweather, 1987, pp. 235-243.
10. Wingate, 1969, 1970; Weiner, 1978.
11. See, e.g., Wingate, 1969; Van Riper, 1982, p. 425; Starkweather, 1987, p. 190.

Part II.

Speech and the Valsalva Mechanism

CHAPTER 4.

The Speech Mechanism

WATCHING THE LIPS of a fluent speaker is a fascinating pastime for someone who stutters. How quickly they move! How lightly they touch! How easy it all seems! What could be the secret?

We know, of course, that speech is a lot more than moving one's lips, or even one's tongue. These are only the most external, visible parts of the speech mechanism. No matter how much effort we put into our lips or tongue, they will not produce speech by themselves. In addition, we need voice, we need airflow. Therefore, to understand the speech mechanism we must go beyond the lips, beyond the mouth, deep into the body itself.

Let's imagine that we can make ourselves very small, and go on our own "fantastic voyage" into the speech mechanism. Like miniature spelunkers, we will explore the caves and tunnels of the mouth, throat, and lungs, to discover the sources of speech.

We begin be climbing through the lips of a fluent speaker. They open, close, purse, and widen, as if gently caressing the words as they emerge. We need not fear being injured, because the lips do not close tightly, but gently and briefly, as in a casual kiss.

Behind the lips are the teeth. Even as we climb between the upper and lower incisors, we don't feel threatened. There is no biting or clenching of the teeth. The jaw moves gently, in a relaxed manner. We can feel the air flowing through.

After sliding down the back of the teeth, we are suddenly overwhelmed by a giant, fleshy mass that constantly moves and undulates and changes shape. It is the tongue. We notice how the tip of the tongue sometimes touches the tips of the upper teeth. Sometimes it touches the teeth ridge, or gums, above the teeth. Sometimes the middle of the tongue rises up to meet the roof of the mouth, which is called the **hard palate**. For a thrill, we might want to sit on the tongue and ride it. We may get bounced around a bit, but we are not pressed against anything hard enough or long enough to get hurt.

As we move to the back of the mouth, we turn on our headlamps, since it is now quite dark. Above us is the **soft palate**. This is a muscular extension of the palate, which ends in the **uvula** — that cone-shaped projection you see hanging down at the back of the mouth. The soft palate can move up and down, to either close or open the passageway between the nasal cavity and the upper part of the throat, called the **pharynx**.

At the back of tongue, we fasten our climbing gear to keep from sliding down into the pharynx. We shine our lights into the deep pit and see that there is a fork in the tunnel. Toward the back is the food tube, called the **esophagus**, which leads to the stomach. Not wanting to be digested, we take the branch to the front, which is the windpipe. We hear a loud buzzing sound coming from this direction.

Directly below us is an enlargement in the windpipe, called the **larynx**. It is an oddly shaped box of cartilage and muscles, which is constantly moving in various ways. At the top is a tongue-shaped lid, the **epiglottis**. This closes off the top of the larynx during swallowing, to prevent food

Chapter 4 / The Speech Mechanism

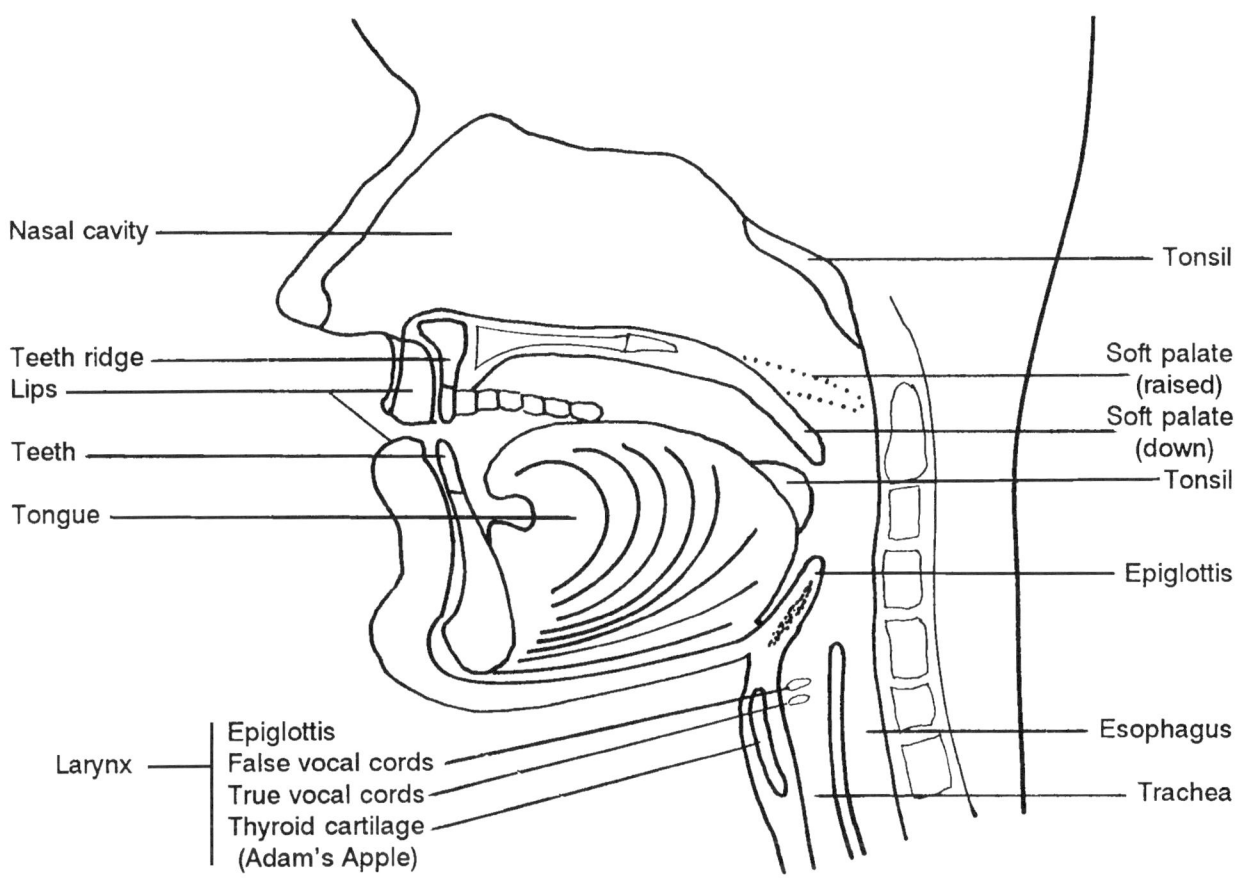

THE MOUTH AND AIRWAY

from accidentally going down the windpipe. During speech, it is open.

We go into the larynx and pass between two protrusions, called the **false vocal cords** or **vestibular folds**. Below them is a fascinating sight. We see what appear to be two lips, which are anchored together at the front and which open and close at the back. These are the **true vocal cords**, or **vocal folds**. (Although "vocal folds" is now the scientifically accepted term, we shall continue to call them "vocal cords," as they are popularly known.) Their posterior ends — those toward the back — are attached to two small pieces of cartilage, called the **arytenoid cartilages**, which swing open and closed like a little gate. When the vocal cords are open, the opening (called the **glottis**) is V-shaped. When they are closed, the glottis is reduced to just a slit.

The vocal cords seem to open and close almost instantaneously. While they are open, there is no sound — just the rush of air from below. When they are in the closed position, they still leave a tiny slit for the air to come through. As it does, it causes the vocal cords to ripple and vibrate, which creates the buzzing sound we hear. This sound is called **phonation**.

There are certain tiny muscles in the larynx that move the vocal cords together, and others that move them apart. During speech, the vocal cords rapidly open and close to turn the voice on and off, depending on whether a voiced or unvoiced sound is being made. Other muscles are involved in adjusting the pitch of the voice. This is done by moving the larynx in such a way as to increase or decrease tension of the vocal cords. However, the actual vibration of the vocal cords is not caused by muscular activity, but rather by the airflow passing between them.

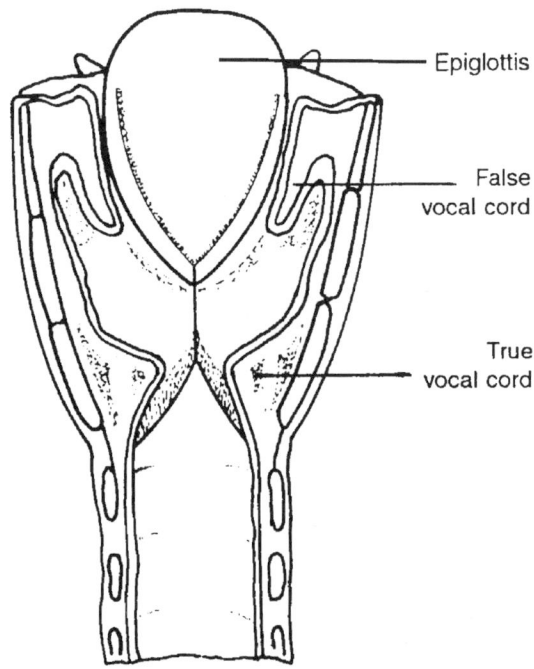

FRONTAL-SECTION OF THE LARYNX

Where is the air coming from? While the vocal cords are open, we quickly drop through. Now we are in the **windpipe**, or **trachea**. We come to a fork in the tunnel, with branches going left and right. These are the **bronchi**, which lead to the left and right lungs. The lungs are soft, spongy, elastic, cone-shaped organs. It is here that life-giving oxygen is transferred into the blood and carbon dioxide is removed.

We notice that the lungs repeatedly expand and contract. As they expand, air rushes down the windpipe into the lungs. As the lungs contract, the air rushes up the windpipe, through the larynx, and out the mouth. It is this outward flow of air that powers our speech. But what exactly causes the air to flow? To understand this, we must know something about the mechanics of breathing.

The lungs, together with the heart, are located in the **thoracic** or **chest cavity**. This is the space within the chest, surrounded by the rib cage. Just below the lungs is a thin, wide muscle called the **diaphragm**. This separates the chest cavity from the **abdominal cavity**, which contains the stomach, liver, intestines, and other organs.

When the diaphragm is relaxed, it is shaped like a dome — its center arching upward under the lungs and heart. But when the muscle fibers in the diaphragm tense up and contract, the diaphragm flattens out. In effect, the center of the diaphragm moves downward. This has two results — it causes the chest cavity to become larger and the abdominal cavity to become smaller. It squeezes down on the stomach, intestines, and other organs.

The lungs are like balloons. As the chest cavity becomes larger, the surface of the lungs sticks to the inner wall of the chest cavity, causing the lungs to expand also. As the space in the lungs increases, air is sucked down the windpipe and into the lungs.

This is the process of inhaling — sometimes called **inspiration**. When a person inhales by using the diaphragm, it is called **diaphragmatic breathing** or **abdominal breathing**. Another way in which people inhale is called **chest breathing**. Certain muscles in the chest (the **external intercostal muscles**) contract, moving the rib cage upward and outward. As the rib cage rises, this also expands the size of the chest cavity, causing the lungs to expand and to draw air in.

You can tell if a person is chest breathing, because you can see his chest rising as he inhales and falling as he exhales. You can tell if he's using the diaphragm to breathe, because his abdomen will protrude as he inhales, since the diaphragm pushes down on the intestines, etc., causing them to bulge outward in front. The abdomen then goes back in as he exhales. Typically, a person will use both the diaphragm and the chest muscles while inhaling.

Inhalation, or inspiration, is the only part of breathing that requires muscular activity. Exhaling, or **expiration**, does not require activation of any muscles. It all can be done by simply relaxing the same muscles that were used for inhaling. The chest muscles relax and the rib cage lowers. The diaphragm relaxes and the abdominal organs push

TOP VIEW OF THE VOCAL CORDS

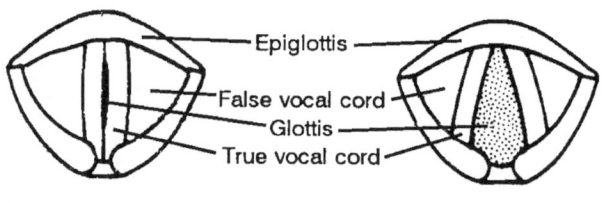

CLOSED   OPEN

Chapter 4 / The Speech Mechanism

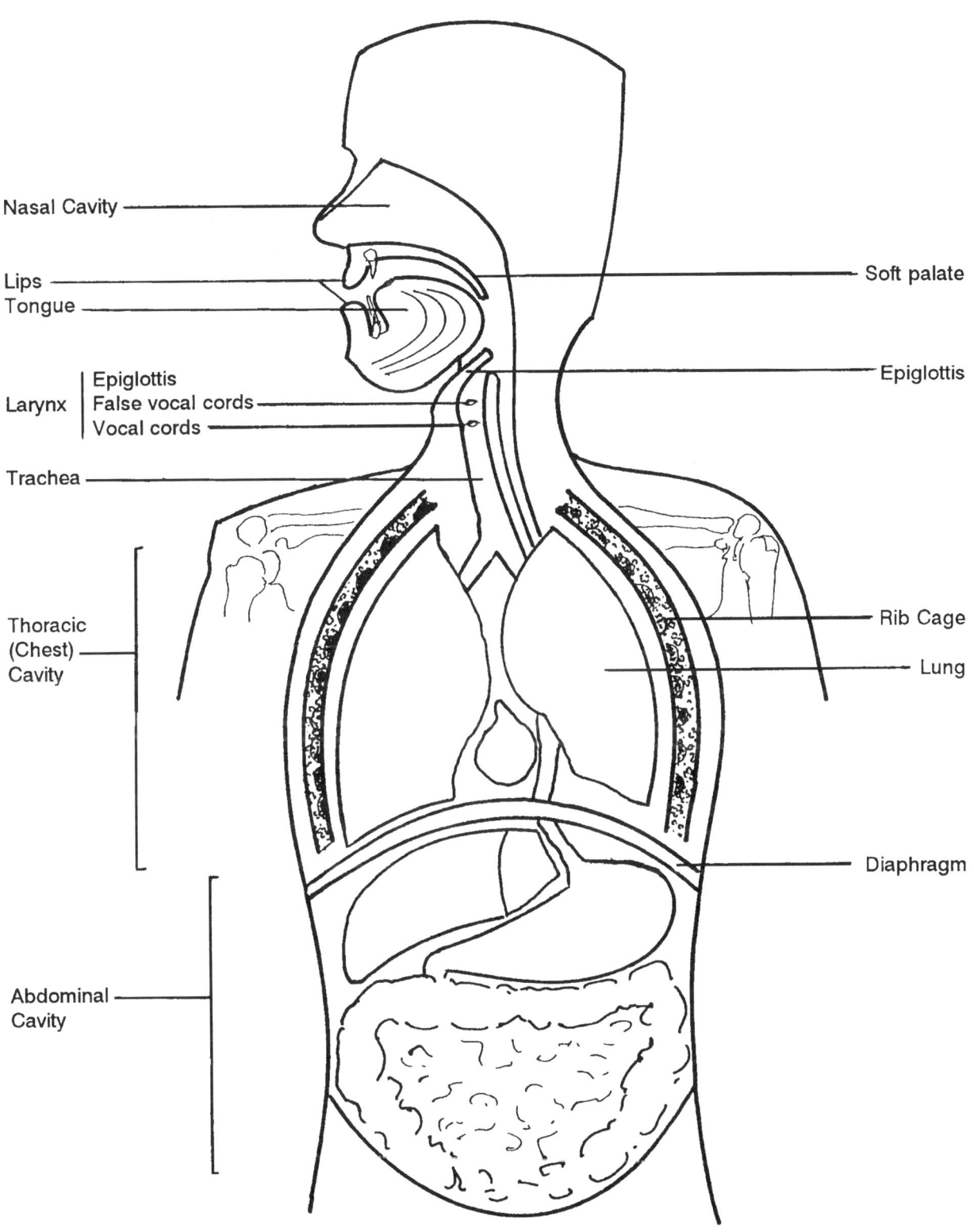

THE SPEECH MECHANISM

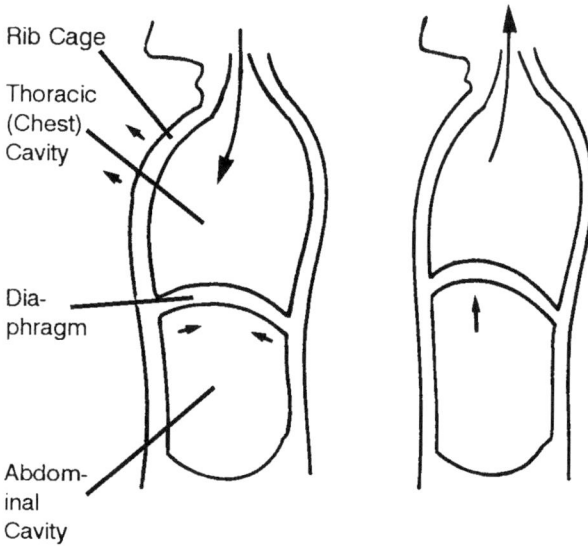

INSPIRATION   EXPIRATION

it back upward into its dome-shaped position. The lungs then contract because of their own elasticity — just as a balloon gets smaller when you let the air out.

What significance does this have for speech? In the English language, all speech occurs while we *exhale*. Therefore, *speech does not require much muscular effort for airflow*. While respiratory muscles normally help to maintain appropriate levels of air pressure, it is theoretically possible to speak with **passive airflow**, the air that naturally flows out *while we relax*.

Of course, one can also force the air out of the lungs. This is called **forced expiration**. However, this is not usually needed unless we are exercising vigorously, blowing a trumpet, or inflating a balloon. In forced expiration, other muscles in the chest (the **internal intercostal muscles**) contract, drawing the ribs closer together and compressing the chest cavity. In addition, the muscles around the abdominal cavity may also tighten up, squeezing the intestines and other organs, forcing them upward against the diaphragm, pushing it higher into the chest cavity. This increases the air pressure in the lungs, causing the air to be squeezed out.

The use of the abdominal muscles to force out air should not be confused with using the diaphragm. The diaphragm only contracts during inhalation. It relaxes during exhalation. The abdominal muscles, on the other hand, tighten for the purpose of increasing air pressure in the lungs, so as to force the air out. In normal speech, this effort is usually not very noticeable, unless we are shouting or singing loudly.

Now that we have explored the depths of the speech mechanism, we will next examine how all of these parts work together in the production of speech.

General References

CARLSON, A. J., JOHNSON, V., & CAVERT, H. M. *The Machinery of the Body.* Chicago: University of Chicago Press, 1961, pp. 252-262.

DENES, P. B. & PINSON, E. N. *The Speech Chain.* New York: W.H. Freeman & Co., 1993.

DICKSON, D. R., & MAUE-DICKSON, W. *Anatomical and Physiological Bases of Speech.* Boston: Little, Brown & Co., 1982.

FINK, B. R. *The Human Larynx: A Functional Study.* New York: Raven Press, 1975.

FINK, B. R., & DEMAREST, R. *Laryngeal Biomechanics.* Cambridge, Mass: Harvard University Press, 1978.

GRAY, H. *Anatomy of the Human Body.* Philadelphia: Lea & Febiger, 1959.

LADEFOGED, P. Linguistic aspects of respiratory phenomena. *Annals of New York Academy of Sciences,* 1968, 155, 141-151.

CHAPTER 5.

The Basics of Speech

SPEECH IS THE PROCESS of turning thoughts into sound. We choose the ideas we want to express. We select the appropriate words to convey those ideas. We know how those words are supposed to sound. Now we must use all the parts of our speech mechanism, described in the previous chapter, to make those sounds. But how?

Viewed most simply, the production of speech involves three basic elements: **airflow, phonation,** and **articulation**.

Airflow

In the previous chapter, we examined how our breathing apparatus produces the airflow that powers our speech. Breathing has two basic steps: *inhaling* (or inspiration) and *exhaling* (or expiration). Before we can speak, we must first inhale to fill our lungs with the air we will need for airflow.

As we learned, inhaling is the only part of breathing that requires muscular activity. When we inhale, the dome-shaped diaphragm, which separates the chest cavity from the abdominal cavity, contracts so that its center moves downward. At the same time, certain muscles in our chest contract, raising the rib cage. Both of these movements cause the chest cavity to increase in size. As the space increases, the pressure of the air in our lungs becomes less than the air outside. As a result, air is sucked into the lungs. While this happens, our larynx remains wide open, letting the air flow in freely.

The airflow of speech is produced by exhaling. When we exhale, our chest muscles and diaphragm slowly relax, allowing the chest cavity and lungs to shrink automatically to their usual size. As the chest cavity becomes smaller, the pressure of the air in the lungs becomes greater than the air outside. Consequently, the air now flows out of the lungs, like air being released from a balloon. The air flows upward through the windpipe and the larynx.

No force, no effort is required in order to exhale. All you need to do is relax. The result, as previously mentioned, is *passive airflow*.

As previously mentioned, it is possible to increase the force of the airflow by contracting our abdominal muscles. These muscles tighten around the intestines and other organs in the abdominal cavity, forcing them upward against the underside of the diaphragm. This pushes the diaphragm higher into the chest cavity, so as to increase the air pressure in the lungs. There is also a set of muscles in the chest which can operate to lower the rib cage, putting additional pressure on the lungs. The result is *forced expiration*.

Phonation

Air rushing out through an open larynx makes very little sound. For voice to be produced, the vocal cords in the larynx must be brought together in such a way that they will vibrate as air passes between them. This vibration is called **phonation**. You can actually *feel* the larynx vibrating by touching your throat, around the Adam's apple, while

As we saw in the previous chapter, the vocal cords are anchored together at their anterior ends

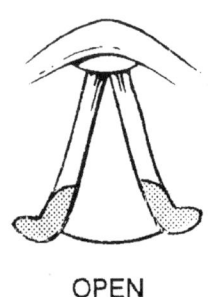 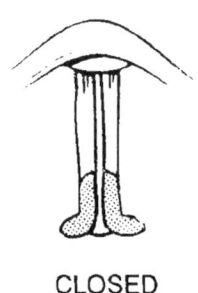

OPEN   CLOSED

VOCAL CORDS AND ARYTENOID CARTILAGES
(SHADED)
(From *The Speech Chain*, by Denes and Pinson.
Copyright © 1993 by W.H. Freeman and Company.
Reprinted with permission.)

— that is, the ends toward the front of the throat. In order for phonation to occur, the posterior ends of the vocal cords must be brought into the closed position. This is done by certain tiny muscles in the larynx that move the arytenoid cartilages together and lock them in position. Other muscles give the vocal cords the proper tension needed for vibration. Still other muscles are used for opening the vocal cords.

For present purposes, it is not necessary to list all these muscles by name. However, it would be helpful if we actually got the feeling of how they operate. Start by making a steady flow of silent breath. Without stopping your breath, turn it into an "aah" sound. Then let your breath be silent again. When you heard your voice, the vocal cords were closed. When the breath was silent, the cords were open.

Did you feel the movement in your larynx? Did you feel the vocal cords as they closed and opened? Continue to practice moving your vocal cords until you become familiar with where they are and how they feel.

During speech, the vocal cords rapidly open and close to turn the voice on and off, depending on whether a voiced or unvoiced sound is being made. The voiced sounds include all of the vowels — *a, e, i, o,* and *u*. Phonation is also needed for most of the consonants — including *b, d, g, j, l, m, n, r, v, w, y,* and *z*.

Some of the consonants are unvoiced; they make use of airflow without phonation. These include the sounds for *c, f, h, k, p, q, s,* and *t*. While these sounds are being made, the vocal cords will open to cut off phonation momentarily.

Then they will close again to give voice to the next part of the word.

It is important to notice that, during normal speech, there is *very little muscular effort* taking place in the larynx. The muscles do not themselves provide the power that makes the vocal cords vibrate. All they do is move the vocal cords in or out of the path of the airflow, and adjust the amount of tension. The vibration is caused by the *airflow*, which is the result of *relaxation* of the chest and diaphragm.

Articulation

As the airflow, now buzzing with phonation, passes up into the pharynx and mouth, it is shaped into the characteristic sounds of the words we are speaking. This shaping process is called **articulation**.

Most articulation is done in the mouth. The **soft palate** — the muscular extension at the back of the hard palate — is usually raised during articulation, thereby blocking off the nasal cavity to keep air from escaping through the nose.

One kind of articulation is the formation of the **vowel sounds**. This is done by changing the size and shape of the mouth cavity by putting the tongue in different positions. It is also affected by the way we shape our lips.

For example, we say "oo" by raising the tongue near the back of the mouth and rounding our lips into a little circle. When we say "ee," the tongue is raised near the front of the mouth and our lips are spread almost into a smile. (This is probably why photographers tell their subjects to say "cheese.") When we say "ah," the tongue is lowered and the lips are open. (Consequently, this is a helpful thing to say when the doctor wants to get a good look at our throat.)

Another kind of articulation involves the various ways in which we create the sounds of **consonants**. Although most people don't give this subject much thought, speech experts have gone to the trouble of classifying each consonant according to the manner in which its sound is made and the parts of the mouth that make it.

A consonant is classified as **labial** if it is made by both lips (such as *p, b, w,* and *m*); **labio-dental** if made by one lip and the teeth (*f* and *v*), **dental** if made by the tongue against the teeth *(th)*; **alveo-**

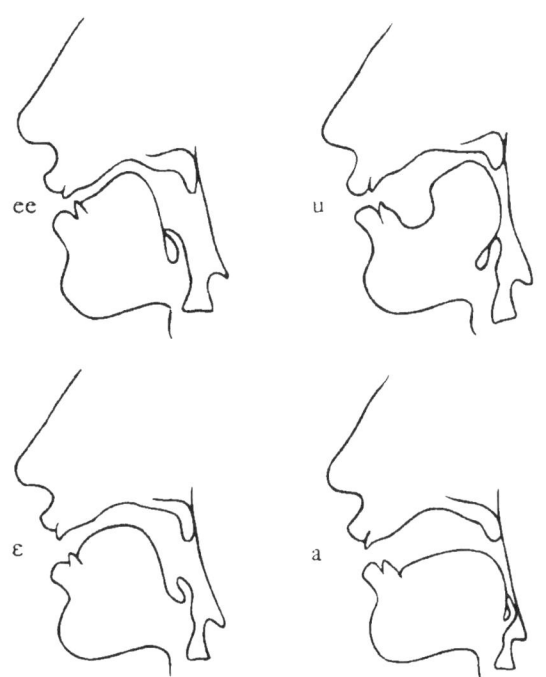

EXAMPLES OF MOUTH POSITIONS FOR VOWELS
(From *The Speech Chain*, by Denes and Pinson. Copyright © 1993 by W.H. Freeman and Company. Reprinted with permission.)

lar if made by the tongue against the gums (*d, t, l, n, r, s, y,* and *z*); **palatal** if made by the tongue against the hard palate (*sh* and *zh*), **velar** if made by the tongue against the soft palate (*k, g,* and *ng*), and **glottal** if made in the larynx (*h*).

As to the manner of articulation, the consonants are classified as **plosive, fricative, liquid, nasal,** and **semi-vowel**.

The **plosive** consonants (*p, b, t, d, k,* and hard *g*) are made by blocking the airflow briefly, so as to let the air pressure build up a little, and then suddenly releasing it in a burst of sound. The blockage may be done by the lips together (as in *p* and *b*), by the tip of the tongue against the upper gums (as in *t* and *d*), or by the back of the tongue against the soft palate (as in *k* and hard *g*).

In making the fricative consonants (*f, v, th, s, z, sh, zh,* and *h*), the airflow is blocked only partially. As the air escapes, this creates a hissing sound if the consonant is unvoiced or a vibrating sound if it is voiced. A distinctively different hiss or vibration is made depending on whether the air passes between the lower lip and the teeth (as in *f* and *v*), the tongue and teeth (*th*), the tongue and gums (*s*

and *z*), or the tongue and the palate (*sh* and *zh*).

Still another kind of hissing sound is made if the constriction takes place, not in the mouth, but in the larynx, as in the sound for *h*. The *h* is an unvoiced sound that is produced while the vocal cords are open and the *false vocal cords* (vestibular folds) are partially closed. This is very similar to what happens when we *whisper*.

The **liquid** consonants (*l* and *r*) are made by placing a part of the tongue against the gums and letting the voiced breath pass through the open space. In making the *l* sound, it is the tip of the tongue that makes contact. In *r*, the sides of the tongue curl up to touch the gums.

The **nasal** consonants (*m, n,* and *ng*) are sounded through the nose. To accomplish this, the soft palate is lowered to permit voiced airflow to pass through the nasal cavity. At the same time, the mouth is closed by the lips *(m)*, by the tongue and gums *(n)*, or by the tongue and soft palate *(ng)*. These are the only consonants in which the soft palate is not raised to block off the nasal cavity.

The **semi-vowels** (*w* and *y*) are made by starting with the mouth in a vowel position and then sliding into the next vowel sound in the word. In making the *w* sound, you start with your mouth in the same position as if you were going to say "oo," and then move right into the vowel that follows it. For example, the mouth position for "wish" is the same as "oo-*ish*," without actually saying the "oo." The *w* sound results when you move from the "oo" position to the next vowel.

In the case of *y*, you start as if you were going to say "ee," and then move to the next vowel. For example, the mouth position for "yard" is like "ee-*ard*."

Not all articulation takes place in the mouth. The larynx is also used to give a plosive effect to vowels that come at the beginning of words — as in *apple*. This type of vowel articulation is known as the **coup de glotte**, or "glottal attack." The vocal cords and false vocal cords momentarily block the airflow, in order to build up air pressure. The air is then suddenly released in a little burst of phonation, which accentuates the beginning of the vowel sound.

During normal speech, there is an overlap in the production of sounds, called **co-articulation**. While one set of muscles is making one sound, another set of muscles is already getting ready to make the next one. Notice, for example, the difference in the shape of your lips when you form the *b* sound in *beet* and in *boot*. In the first instance, the lips are wide, already prepared for the "ee" sound. In the second, they are pursed, ready to form an "oo."

Or try *bat* versus *brat*. In the first, you say the *b* with the tongue flat. In the second, the rear sides of the tongue have already risen in preparation for the *r* sound.

Now we must put all of these elements together: a smooth and easy flow of air; a relaxed larynx, with vocal cords that are ready to close instantly as needed to produce phonation; and a tongue and lips that move gently from one position to the next. Normal speech is just a *sequence of movements*. It requires *very little effort*. Whenever the tongue or lips momentarily block the airflow, they *touch lightly* and *release the air quickly*, without force or struggle, and without building up a lot of air pressure.

If speech should be so easy, why does the stutterer make it so hard? Why does he struggle so violently, press his lips and tongue so forcefully, and build up air pressure until he almost turns purple? Why, in attempting to force the words out, does he do everything in his power to block them in?

Could it be that certain parts of our speech mechanism have *other* biological functions that become activated when the stutterer tries to speak? Might these functions become confused with the speech process in such a way as to make speech so difficult?

Next we will explore just such a possibility.

General References

DENES, P. B. & PINSON, E. N. *The Speech Chain.* New York: W.H. Freeman & Co., 1993.

DICKSON, D. R., & MAUE-DICKSON, W. *Anatomical and Physiological Bases of Speech.* Boston: Little, Brown & Co., 1982.

FINK, B. R. *The Human Larynx: A Functional Study.* New York: Raven Press, 1975.

FINK, B. R., & DEMAREST, R. *Laryngeal Biomechanics.* Cambridge, Mass: Harvard University Press, 1978.

CHAPTER 6.

The Valsalva Mechanism

AS NATURAL AS SPEECH IS to the human species, there is no organ that is devoted exclusively to speaking. The eye is dedicated to seeing, the ear to hearing, the stomach to digesting, and the heart to pumping blood. Speech, on the other hand, requires the interaction of several different parts of the body, all having primary functions other than speaking. The mouth, with its tongue, lips, and teeth, is designed for eating and drinking. The lungs and windpipe are devoted to breathing.

Even the larynx — the voice box itself — is not limited to phonation. It has another function, which has played an important role since the days our ancestors swung from trees. The larynx helps us perform acts of *strenuous physical effort*.

To demonstrate what I mean by this, let's start with an exercise.

Stand up. Curl your fingers, and link both hands together in front of your chest. Take a deep breath. Now try to pull your hands apart, as hard as you can, without letting go.[1] Pull really hard. Now relax.

What did you notice while you were pulling? Obviously, the muscles in your arms and hands were tense. Your chest and shoulders were rigid. You may have also noticed that the muscles in your chest and abdomen, all down the front of your body, were tight. But what else was happening?

Try the same exercise again. Take another deep breath, pull as hard as you can, and this time pay attention to your *throat*. If you are like most people, you will notice that your throat is not only tense, but *it is completely closed*. Furthermore, the harder you pull, the more tightly your throat squeezes shut.

Now try to feel *where* in your throat this closure is occurring. You'll find that it's happening right behind your Adam's Apple, in the same place where your voice is produced — the *larynx*.

The larynx is doing one of the basic tasks for which it is designed. It is called **effort closure**. It is the body's way of closing the upper end of the windpipe, in order to keep air in the lungs.[2]

During effort closure, the muscles of the larynx behave much differently than they do during phonation. Phonation is produced by bringing the vocal cords gently together, while a stream of air passes between them. This causes the vocal folds to vibrate, creating the sound of our voice. Meanwhile, the false vocal cords (vestibular folds), which are located above the vocal cords, remain open.

CROSS-SECTION OF THE LARYNX
(From Fink & Demarest, 1978)

False Vocal Cords   False Vocal Cords

Vocal Cords   Vocal Cords

PHONATION   EFFORT CLOSURE

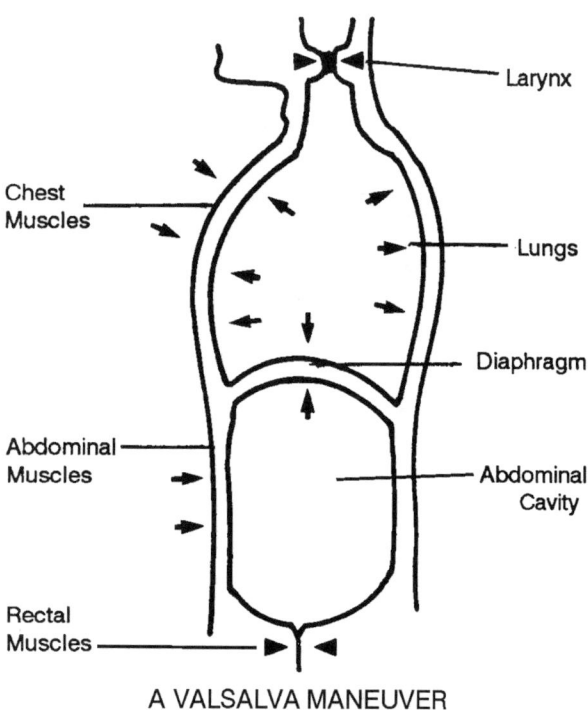

A VALSALVA MANEUVER

Effort closure, on the other hand, is accomplished by pressing both the false vocal cords and the vocal cords tightly together. The inside of the larynx squeezes shut, like a fist, totally blocking the airway.[3] The larynx is designed to close with enough force to hold back any amount of air pressure that may come from the lungs.

Now repeat the hand-pulling exercise, and pay closer attention to what the rest of the body is doing. Notice the tension in your *chest muscles*. They are straining to pull your rib cage downward, in order to put pressure on your lungs.

How about your *abdominal muscles* — the ones across the front of your body, below the belt? Do you notice how they have tightened up? These muscles are squeezing against the intestines and other organs in your abdominal cavity, forcing them upward against your diaphragm. As the center of the diaphragm is pushed upward, it also puts greater pressure on your lungs.

And what about your *lungs*? Do they feel as if they're going to burst? It's no wonder. Your chest and abdominal muscles are doing everything they can to force air out of your lungs. At the same time, your larynx is straining equally as hard to keep the air blocked in. As a result, the air pressure in the lungs becomes greater and greater.

What is going on? And why?

You are performing a **Valsalva maneuver**. This is a normal bodily function that occurs in all healthy human beings when they exert strenuous physical effort.[4] Although most people never give it a thought, the Valsalva maneuver has been known to medical science for more than two hundred years. It takes its name from Anton Maria Valsalva, an Italian anatomist who lived from 1666 to 1723.

When we do a Valsalva maneuver, we block our upper airway while we tighten our chest and abdominal muscles to put pressure on our lungs. This has the same effect as squeezing a partially inflated balloon. At first the balloon feels soft, but as we increase the air pressure by squeezing, the balloon feels harder and harder. When we do the Valsalva maneuver, it is like pressurizing a balloon inside our chest.

Pressurized air can give strength and rigidity. We are all familiar with those inflatable rubber toys, which are soft and limp when there isn't much air in them. But when we blow them up with plenty of air, they become rigid; they stand up and hold their shape. A flat tire can't do very much. But when it's filled with pressurized air, it can support an automobile weighing thousands of pounds. Likewise, our body is firmer, more rigid, and can exert effort more efficiently when we pressurize our lungs by doing a Valsalva maneuver.

Have you ever noticed how a weight lifter "holds his breath" as he strains to raise a heavy bar bell over his head? He is doing a Valsalva maneuver. The air pressure in his lungs keeps his chest and shoulders firm and rigid, giving greater support to his arms. In this way, he can direct all his energy toward lifting the weight. Otherwise, some of that energy would be wasted as his chest and shoulders sagged.

By using the Valsalva maneuver, we brace and stiffen the trunk of our bodies. This helps our arms and legs perform many kinds of strenuous tasks, such as lifting, pushing, pulling, rowing, climbing, and pressing downward with our feet. The next time you perform any of these activities, notice how your larynx instinctively closes up. You are doing a Valsalva maneuver.

This does not mean that you *must* use the Valsalva maneuver when you exert effort. If you consciously think about it, you can tell your body *not* to close the larynx while you are pulling, lifting, etc. The Valsalva maneuver just helps us to do those jobs more forcefully.

The Valsalva maneuver can also help us perform other kinds of bodily functions, such as defecation, urination, and childbirth.[5] In these activities, we tighten our abdominal muscles in an effort to squeeze various things out of our abdominal cavity. The larynx naturally closes up, to keep air in the lungs. The resulting air pressure helps to stabilize the diaphragm, so that the abdominal pressure will be directed downward more efficiently. This activity most commonly occurs when a person tries to force out a bowel movement.

Again, the Valsalva maneuver is not absolutely necessary for defecation. You can consciously choose to keep your larynx open, if you wish.[6] There are other muscles inside the abdomen that are capable of moving the bowels on their own. The Valsalva maneuver simply allows us to apply additional downward force, in an effort to help the job along.

When defecation is intended, the **rectal** and **anal muscles** relax, thereby permitting the bowel movement to be expelled. However, when defecation is *not* intended, these muscles tighten up during the Valsalva maneuver, to prevent an accidental evacuation of the bowels. The principal safeguard is the **puborectalis muscle**. It forms a sling around the **rectum** — the tube that carries waste material from the intestines to the anus. When the puborectalis muscle tightens, it chokes off the rectum to keep anything from escaping.[7]

You can confirm this yourself by repeating our previous exercise. This time, as you pull your hands apart, concentrate on your rectum. If you pay careful attention, you will notice that the muscles in that area are tightened up during the Valsalva maneuver.

As a further experiment, voluntarily tighten your anal and rectal muscles. As you did this, did you notice that your larynx automatically closed also?

All of the muscles that we discussed — muscles of the larynx, the chest, the abdomen, and the rectum — are linked together as a "team" by our nervous system. They are neurologically coordinated to contract at the same time in the performance of a Valsalva maneuver. When one of these muscles tightens up, they *all* tighten up — unless we consciously tell them not to. And they all tend to contract with the same degree of force, in proportion to one another.[8]

Therefore, we will refer to this team of muscles as a single, coordinated unit, called the **Valsalva mechanism**. This is the mechanism we use to perform the Valsalva maneuver.

Might this also be a physical mechanism involved in stuttering?

As we discussed in Chapter 3, both the *circumstances* and *symptoms* of stuttering seem to be related to *the exertion of effort*. We tend to stutter more when we feel the need to "try hard" and to use extra effort in speaking. Similarly, stuttering is often characterized by excessive force and effort in the attempt to speak. Therefore, one would expect that the physical mechanism involved in stuttering should have something to do with the exertion of effort and the forceful blockage of airflow. The Valsalva mechanism obviously meets this requirement.

We also observed that stuttering is often characterized by difficulty or delay in phonation. This suggests that the physical mechanism of stuttering must have some effect on the larynx. Again, the Valsalva mechanism qualifies.

As we have seen, the Valsalva mechanism is well-designed to help us exert physical effort and to force out bowel movements. However, it is definitely *not* designed to help us speak or to force out words. On the contrary, it blocks the airflow needed for speech and causes the larynx to tighten up like a fist.

Nevertheless, there is still more to be explained. Thus far, we have only discussed how the *larynx* closes during a Valsalva maneuver. While this might explain stuttering blocks that occur in the larynx, how do we account for stuttering blocks that occur in the *mouth?*

We can quickly solve this mystery by going back to our hand-pulling exercise. Take a deep breath, but before you start pulling your hands apart, put your lips together as if you were saying a *p* sound. Now start pulling your hands apart as hard as you can.

What did you notice about your lips? Most people find that *the lips press tightly together*. The harder you pull your hands, the more forcefully the lips close.

Now see what happens when you press the tip

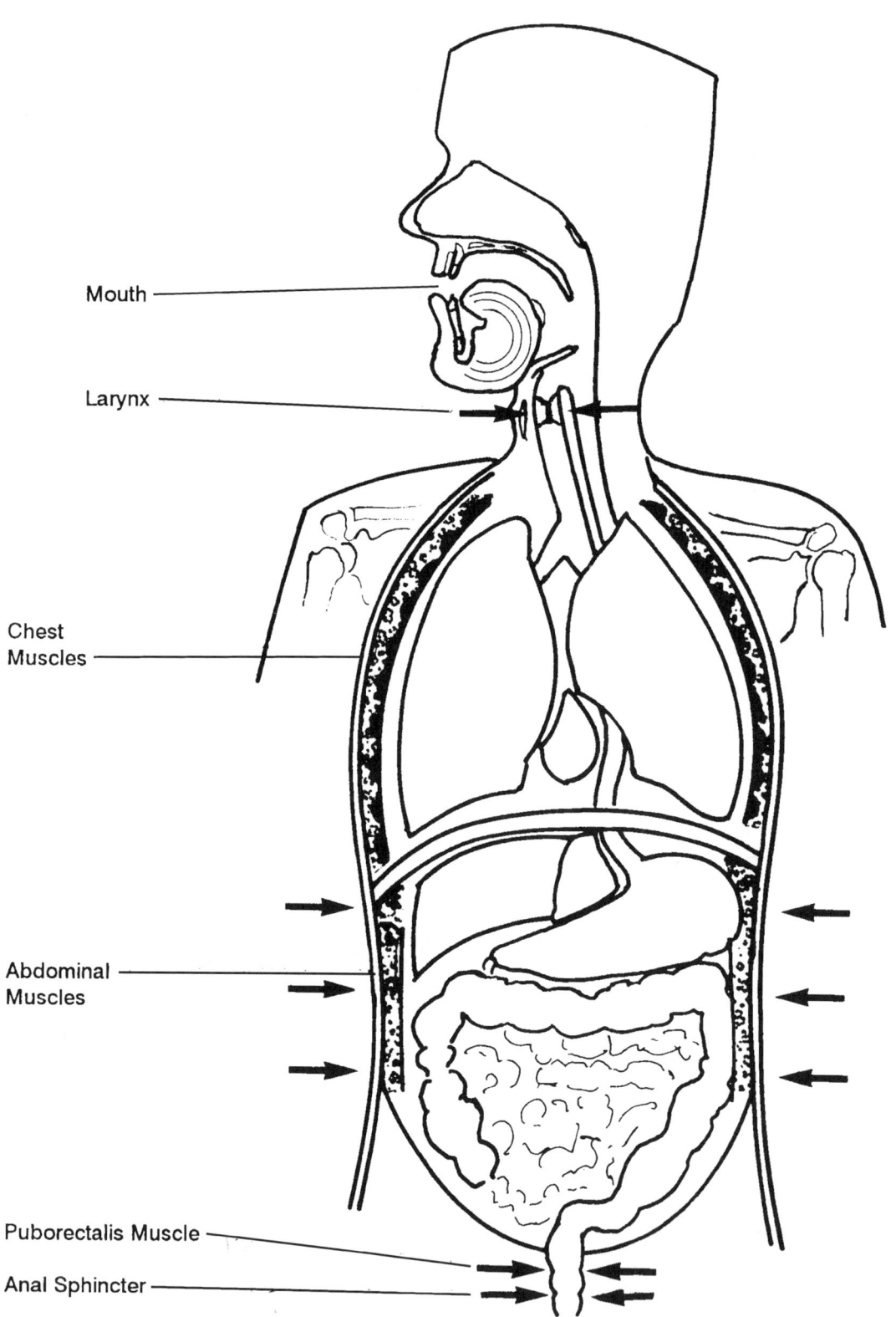

THE VALSALVA MECHANISM

of your tongue to the ridge behind your upper front teeth, as if you were saying the *t* sound. Take a deep breath and start pulling. You will probably find the tip of tongue pressing more and more forcefully.

Finally, touch the back of your tongue to the roof of your mouth, as if you were making the *k* sound. Take a breath and pull again. Now it is the back of your tongue that is pressing forcefully.

Do these forceful closures feel familiar?

In all these instances, you are performing a Valsalva maneuver, but you are using your lips or tongue, rather than the larynx, to keep the air from escaping. The lips and tongue are acting the same as the larynx did, pressing more and more tightly to block the air pressure in the lungs. Therefore, the lips and the tongue can also become part of the Valsalva mechanism.

Whether it will be the lips, tongue, or larynx that performs the closure depends on which one first obstructs the airflow. If you start with your lips closed, then the lips will take over the job of forceful closure during the Valsalva maneuver. Likewise, if some part of the tongue originally stops the airflow, then the same part of the tongue will continue to exert pressure during the Valsalva maneuver. The harder the chest and abdominal muscles try to force the air out, the more forcefully the lips, tongue, or larynx will press, trying to block it in. *The harder you try to break through the closure, the more forceful the closure becomes.* That's what the Valsalva mechanism is all about.

Isn't this remarkably similar to the forceful closures that occur during stuttering?

Is it possible that the Valsalva mechanism somehow becomes activated when a stutterer tries to speak, thereby causing these forceful closures? Might the Valsalva mechanism interfere with speech in other ways as well — such as by inhibiting phonation? These possibilities will be explored in the following chapters.

Notes

See Bibliography for complete citations of references.

1. This exercise is medically known as "Jendrassik's maneuver." Its effect is to stimulate a Valsalva maneuver. Lastovka, 1970.

2. Fink, 1975, pp. 85-100; Fink and Demarest, 1978, pp. 45-63.

3. As noted by Ardram and Kemp, 1967, p. 381, "the larynx is closed from the entrance to the vestibule [false vocal cords] to the level of the vocal folds; the laryngeal ventricles are obliterated." Fink and Demarest, 1978, p. 47, summarize the differences between effort closure and phonation as follows:
"[W]hereas phonatory closure is confined to closure of the glottis, that is, to apposition of the vocal folds by adduction of the arytenoid cartilages, effort closure implicates in addition apposition of the vestibular folds [false vocal cords] and bases of the cuneiform cartilages by the thyroarytenoid muscles, as well as a variable amount of apposition of the median thyrohyoid fold to the top of the adducted vestibular folds."

4. Carlson, Johnson and Cavert, 1961, p. 262; Ardran and Kemp, 1967; Fink, 1973; Fink, 1975, p. 89-92; Fink and Demarest, 1978, pp. 45-63.

5. Dickson and Maue-Dickson, 1982, p. 135.

6. Ardran and Kemp, 1967, p. 381.

7. Fink, 1975, p.99.

8. Fink, 1975, pp. 93-97; Fink and Demarest, 1978, p. 46.

Part III.

The Valsalva Hypothesis

CHAPTER 7.

An Introduction to the Valsalva Hypothesis

WE HAVE SEEN that fluent speech requires very little physical effort. The *airflow* that powers speech comes from the relaxation of our diaphragm and chest muscles. *Phonation* results when we simply close our vocal cords and let airflow pass between them. The *articulation* of words is accomplished by gentle movements of the lips and tongue, which touch lightly and then relax quickly.

In contrast, we have seen that stuttering is often characterized by excessive force and effort in the attempt to speak. Our chest and abdomen may tighten up. Our larynx may squeeze shut. Our lips or tongue may press tightly, stubbornly blocking both airflow and words, as the air pressure and frustration builds up inside us.

We have also seen that there is a bodily mechanism specifically designed to increase air pressure in the lungs, in order to assist us in the exertion of physical effort. This is the **Valsalva mechanism**. It includes muscles of the larynx, chest, abdomen, and rectum that act together to do a **Valsalva maneuver**.

During a Valsalva maneuver, the larynx performs **effort closure** — one of its basic functions other than phonation. The larynx squeezes shut to block our upper airway, while our chest and abdominal muscles tighten to increase the air pressure in our lungs. The pressurized air makes the trunk of our bodies firm and rigid, allowing us to use our arms and legs more efficiently during strenuous physical activities. The Valsalva maneuver also helps us to expel things from our abdominal cavity, as when we force out bowel movements.

As demonstrated in the last chapter, the *mouth* can also be used by the Valsalva mechanism to block the upper airway. A Valsalva maneuver can cause forceful closures by the *lips* and *tongue*, similar to the blockages that we experience during stuttering.

In trying to figure out my own stuttering problem, I became intrigued by the similarities between the forceful closures of stuttering and the Valsalva maneuver. During severe blocks, my mouth or larynx would clamp shut, while my abdominal and chest muscles would contract, as if straining to force air through the closure. However, the closure would just tighten more than ever. This seemed identical to what happens during a Valsalva maneuver.

As I studied my behavior more carefully, I noticed that my stuttering (even when less severe) was preceded and accompanied by tension in certain muscles in and around the larynx, the abdomen, and the rectum — all of which are connected with the Valsalva mechanism. I noted that I had difficulties or delays in initiating phonation, which also involves the larynx, a part of the same mechanism. Could it be that the Valsalva mechanism was somehow involved in my stuttering?

A Fiber-Optic View of the Larynx

One of the first things I wanted to verify was the similarity between the larynx's behavior during a Valsalva maneuver and during a stuttering block. My stuttering on initial vowel sounds (such as the *a* in *apple*) involved tight closure of the larynx. To me, this felt exactly the same as the effort closure done by the larynx during a Valsalva maneuver.

To get an actual view of my larynx at work, I obtained the help of Dr. Joseph P. Atkins, Jr., Chief of Otolaryngology at the Pennsylvania Hospital in Philadelphia. His department was equipped with a **fiberoptic nasopharyngoscope** — a sophisticated instrument designed for viewing the larynx without interfering with the movement of the mouth.

The device consisted of a long, flexible tube, containing hundreds of tiny glass fibers. A miniature camera lens focused an image onto one end of the bundle of fibers. The fibers carried individual dots of light to the other end of the tube, where they formed a picture. This was photographed by a television camera, displayed on a color TV monitor, and videotaped.

The fiberoptic tube was inserted through the nose, snaked up through the nasal cavity, and then lowered down through the pharynx, behind the back of the tongue. Light from the tube illuminated the inside of the larynx as it was photographed. Meanwhile, I sat back in a chair and watched the TV pictures, as Dr. Atkins explained what was happening.

We could clearly see the arytenoid cartilages, which control the opening and closing of not only the V-shaped vocal cords, but also the false vocal cords located above them. When I held my breath, as in a Valsalva maneuver, the arytenoid cartilages clamped together, tightly closing the false vocal cords to block the air. This was the larynx performing effort closure.

When I blocked on an initial vowel sound, the larynx looked exactly as it did during effort closure. Again the arytenoid cartilages were clamped together and the false vocal cords were blocking the air. When I stuttered repetitively on a vowel sound ("uh-uh-uh-uh-uh-uh"), we could see the arytenoid cartilages and false vocal cords rapidly opening and closing.

The closure of the larynx was not as complete when I used my mouth to block the air. I pressed my lips together to resist the air pressure during a Valsalva maneuver. The larynx closed somewhat, but not tightly enough to shut the airway. The same was true when I blocked on consonants in the mouth during stuttering. Although the larynx did not completely close, the arytenoid cartilages clearly jerked together at each stuttering block. The larynx seemed to be acutely sensitive to the stuttering blocks, even though the actual closure was taking place in the mouth.

The fiber-optic study also gave me a firsthand view of how the various parts of the Valsalva mechanism interact with one another. For example, whenever I tightened my rectal muscles or my abdominal muscles, I could see the larynx automatically respond by closing tightly. Conversely, when I relaxed my rectum, the pictures showed the larynx in a relaxed, open position.

Neuromotor Tuning

Now that I had confirmed, to my satisfaction, the similarities between the forceful closures of stuttering and those of the Valsalva maneuver, my next question was *how* the Valsalva mechanism might interfere with the process of speech. It seemed possible that there might be, under certain circumstances, some kind of neurological confusion between the speech and the Valsalva mechanism. I wondered how such a confusion might take place.

During my research in the medical libraries, I learned some interesting facts about how our nervous system prepares our muscles for movement.

Movement takes place by the contraction of muscles. The muscles contain fibers that **contract** — or shorten in length — when they become activated. When the muscle fibers are relaxed or "turned off," they return to their usual, longer length. An individual muscle fiber will contract completely, or not at all.[1] The strength with which the entire muscle contracts depends on how many of the individual fibers are contracting at the same time.

The muscle fibers are controlled by nerve cells called **motor neurons**, which receive impulses from the **central nervous system** (the brain and spinal cord) telling the muscle fibers when to contract. Each motor neuron controls a group of muscle fibers, called a **motor unit**. As in the case of muscle fibers, activation of each individual motor neuron is an "all or nothing" proposition.[2]

Whether or not an individual neuron becomes activated depends largely on its **excitability** to the impulses it receives (also called its **threshold level**). In other words, the neuron is "set" to react to impulses of a certain strength. If the excitability of the neuron is low, it will be less likely to respond

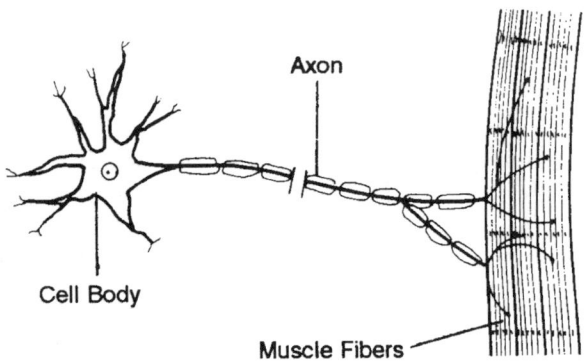

SIMPLIFIED VIEW OF A MOTOR NEURON

to an impulse, and therefore the muscle fibers will remain at rest. On the other hand, if the neuron is very excitable, it is more likely to stimulate a muscular contraction.

There are other types of nerve cells, called **sensory neurons**, which pick up various sensations (including movement, pressure, etc.) through receptors in the skin or other parts of the body. These neurons also behave on the "all or nothing" principle. When the strength of the stimulus reaches the neuron's threshold level, the neuron sends an impulse to the central nervous system.

Scientific studies have revealed that all physical activity (including speech) is preceded by neurological **tuning** of the excitability of all the motor and sensory neurons and nerve pathways that will be involved in performing the particular movement.[3] This usually occurs a fraction of a second before the **triggering impulse** that actually signals the beginning of the movement. By means of this tuning, the central nervous system is able to designate, in advance, which combination of nerves and muscles will act together as a "team" to perform the desired motion.

The tuning makes some of the neurons more excitable, and others less excitable, to the triggering impulse that is to follow. It is as if the nervous system says to some neurons, "Pay attention! Get ready to contract your motor unit when the next command comes!" To others it says, "Relax. Disregard the next command, because it's not meant for you." A fraction of a second later, the triggering command comes down the line: "Go!" The neurons and their motor units either respond or don't respond, depending on their level of excitability.

You can demonstrate this principle yourself, by playing this trick on your friends. First show them how, by contracting different muscle groups, you can make your hand into a fist, or do other things such as pointing a finger. Then tell your friends to make fist, as fast as they can, when you say "Now!"

"Get ready to make a fist," you warn them. Then say, "Now!" as you make a fist yourself. "Not bad," you tell them, "but you're not doing it fast enough. Let's try again."

Repeat this exercise a few times, so that everyone has gotten into the habit of making a fist as fast as they can. Then, after again instructing them, "Get ready to make fist," suddenly say, "*Point*," and point your finger. I have found that most people will reflexively make a fist instead — because that is what their nerves and muscles are ready to do.

This process of neuromotor tuning may be a key to understanding the possible confusion between speech and the Valsalva mechanism. For various reasons, a person's nerves and muscles might become neurologically tuned for a Valsalva maneuver rather than for speech, resulting in forceful closures and other kinds of stuttering behavior.

The Valsalva Hypothesis

When scientists try to understand a phenomenon, they often begin by formulating a **working hypothesis**. This is a tentative explanation, arrived at through logical reasoning, that seems to fit whatever facts are already known about the subject. The scientists then use this hypothesis as a focal point for further research. They plan experiments and other studies designed to test whether the hypothesis is true or false. After analyzing the results of their experiments, they may confirm the hypothesis to be true, or they might have to modify it or discard it altogether. In any event, this method helps to increase the scientists' knowledge about the problem they are studying.

We are now ready to formulate our own working hypothesis about stuttering — one that we can test and modify through our own experience. We will call it the **Valsalva Hypothesis**.[4] We can start out very generally and add details later. Briefly stated, this hypothesis proposes the following:

Stuttering is an interference with speech that

may result from a neurological confusion between speech and the Valsalva mechanism.

The speech mechanism of a person who stutters has the basic capability of fluent speech. Under certain circumstances, however, the person's nerves and muscles become neurologically tuned for a Valsalva maneuver, rather than for speech. The degree of such tuning might be influenced by psychological and emotional factors, and would more likely occur in those instances when the person feels a particular need to "try hard" to get the words out.

The tuning of the Valsalva mechanism would increase the excitability of those nerves and muscles to stimuli that would trigger a Valsalva maneuver. One such stimulus might be the abrupt increase in air pressure that occurs at the beginning of articulation.[5] (This will be discussed more fully in the next chapter.) The Valsalva mechanism would then become activated, causing involuntary muscular contractions in the mouth or larynx to block the upper airway.

Even when forceful closures do not occur, it is possible that the tuning of the Valsalva mechanism might interfere with phonation in the larynx. For example, if the larynx were neurologically prepared for effort closure, it would not be ready to phonate. This would result in a delay in speaking while the larynx became re-tuned for phonation.

It should be emphasized that the Valsalva Hypothesis merely suggests a possible explanation for certain stuttering *behaviors* — in particular, those involving the excessively forceful closures of the mouth or larynx or difficulties in phonation that are common to most people who stutter. It simply focuses on one important piece of the stuttering puzzle, while recognizing that a variety of other factors may also influence stuttering in different individuals.

We also recognize that the common definition of "stuttering" is so broad that it is often applied to disfluencies not characterized by forceful closures or difficulties in phonation. Even if the Valsalva Hypothesis does not apply to these particular cases, it may still be relevant to the great majority of people who stutter.

We will next explore, in greater detail, the various ways in which neuromotor tuning of the Valsalva mechanism might interfere with speech and result in some of the principal kinds of stuttering behavior.

Notes

See Bibliography for complete citation of references.

1. Hole, 1981, p. 226.

2. Brooks, 1986; Tortora and Anagnostakos, 1981.

3. Zimmerman, Smith, and Hanley, 1981; Brooks, 1986, pp. 111-128.

4. Parry, 1985b.

5. Starkweather, 1987, pp. 39-44.

CHAPTER 8.

Valsalva Tuning and the Stuttering Block

THE CRUCIAL MOMENT that determines fluency or stuttering is the split second before a word is spoken. Within this fraction of a second, our brain sends nerve impulses to the motor neurons that control the muscles of the mouth, larynx, and respiratory system, preparing them for the production of speech.

Through the process of **neuromotor tuning**, the brain adjusts the excitability of the motor neurons, so that some will be more sensitive, and others less sensitive, to various stimuli that will come later. If we are to be fluent, the appropriate muscles of the speech mechanism must be "tuned up," so they will be ready to react quickly to the **triggering signals** that the brain sends out when speech begins. Conversely, the muscles of the Valsalva mechanism must be "tuned down," so they will remain inactive and not interfere with speech.

In the last chapter, we introduced the hypothesis that some kinds of stuttering might result because of a *confusion in neuromotor tuning*. Rather than tuning our speech mechanism for speech, our brain might instead tune our Valsalva mechanism for the performance of a *Valsalva maneuver* — a bodily function that blocks the upper airway in order to build up air pressure in the lungs.

Because the Valsalva mechanism is designed to assist us in exerting physical effort and in forcing things out of the body, we might have a tendency to "tune up" the Valsalva mechanism when we anticipate difficulty in speaking, in the mistaken belief that it will help us "force" the words out. However, if our body is tuned for a Valsalva maneuver, it will *not* be ready for speech when the triggering signals come. On the contrary, it will be ready to do things that make fluent speech impossible.

The two principal ways in which Valsalva tuning might interfere with speech are by: (1) promoting forceful closures of the mouth or larynx that block airflow; and (2) inhibiting phonation. Both of these problems may combine to cause different types of stuttering, as we shall discuss in later chapters. For the moment, however, we shall concentrate on the first of these two elements. Let's begin by examining how Valsalva tuning might result in the excessively forceful closures of a full-blown stuttering block.

Anatomy of a Block

Imagine that you have been invited to a dinner party. You are seated at a long table, surrounded by people you hope to impress. Although you are afraid of stuttering, you would like someone to pass the potatoes, which are at the other end of the table.

If you were a normal speaker, you would simply say, "Pass the potatoes, please." But you have been having trouble with your *p*'s lately, and this short sentence presents one hurdle after another. Nevertheless, you muster your courage, take a deep breath, and give it a try.

What is *supposed* to happen at this point? Your chest muscles and diaphragm should relax, allowing your lungs to contract naturally, releasing a gentle flow of air through your larynx and mouth. To form the *p*, your lips should close, momentarily blocking the airflow in order to build up a little air pressure. Then the lips are supposed to relax, releasing a puff of air, which makes the *p* sound.

How do the lips know when to open? One possible explanation is that the increase in air pressure is sensed by pressure-sensitive nerve endings (called **mechanoreceptors**) found in the lower part of the larynx and elsewhere along the respiratory tract.[1] They would stimulate sensory neurons to send impulses to the brain, indicating the amount of air pressure. When just enough pressure has been built up, the brain would signal the lips to let go.

That is what is *supposed* to happen. Now let's see what might go wrong, according to the Valsalva Hypothesis.

In the split second before you exhale and begin speaking, things start to go haywire. Your brain, realizing that a dreaded *p* word is coming, starts to panic. Whether consciously or unconsciously, your mind anticipates that *saying the word will be difficult*. It decides that extra effort will be needed to get over the hurdle. Suddenly, you are overcome by an urge to "try hard" to force the word out.

Your brain sends an S.O.S. to the Valsalva mechanism. "We need help! Get ready to force!"

All the nerves and muscles of the Valsalva mechanism now become neurologically tuned to a high degree of excitability. They are geared up to perform a Valsalva maneuver the instant a triggering signal, or stimulus, comes down the line. Depending on the degree of excitability, almost anything might set them off. One kind of triggering stimulus could be the increase in air pressure that normally occurs during articulation.

A perfect example is the air pressure that builds up when you close your lips to say the letter *p*. As mentioned before, the increased air pressure causes mechanoreceptors to send nerve impulses to the brain. Normally, these impulses would tell the lips when to open. However, if the Valsalva mechanism is overly excitable, these impulses could have just the *opposite* effect. The increased air pressure could be misinterpreted as *the beginning of a Valsalva maneuver* — triggering a responsive reaction by the entire Valsalva mechanism.

As we have seen, the Valsalva mechanism cares nothing about the complexities of speech. It has but one purpose: *to increase air pressure in the lungs*, which it does by squeezing the chest and abdomen while forcefully closing the upper airway. Therefore, the signals from the mechanoreceptors would stimulate the lips *to close more tightly*, to keep the air from escaping.

At the same time, your chest and abdominal muscles would be stimulated to contract, to increase the lung pressure even more. Across your chest, certain muscles would draw the ribs together and downward, compressing the chest cavity. This would create the sensation of the chest tightening up, or a great weight pressing down on the chest, which has been reported by many stutterers. The abdominal muscles would also tighten, as well as the rectal muscles. The trunk of your body would be tense all over.

As the chest and abdominal muscles squeezed, the air pressure in your lungs would continue to rise. The increased air pressure would further stimulate the mechanoreceptors. They would send more signals to the brain, which would, in turn, stimulate the lips to close with proportionately greater force, to resist the increased pressure coming from the lungs. The result would be a vicious cycle, making fluent speech impossible for as long as the maneuver continued.

Blocking on Plosives

The same type of blocking might be stimulated by the articulation of any sound that requires the momentary obstruction of airflow and a resulting increase in air pressure. Whichever part of the mouth starts the closure during articulation — the lips or tongue — will be the part that continues the forceful closure during the Valsalva maneuver.

The Valsalva hypothesis would therefore provide a clue as to why stutterers have particular difficulty with *plosive* consonants (such as *b*, hard *c, d,* hard *g, k, p,* and *t*), which require a complete blockage of airflow during their articulation. It may explain why stuttering is more frequent at the *beginnings of words* and on *stressed syllables*[2] — instances in which abrupt increases in air pressure are most likely.[3] It may also explain why stuttering is often reduced when the speaker uses a "gentle onset" of voice and "light contacts" in articulation, since such methods would tend to avoid abrupt increases in air pressure.

Stuttering blocks can also occur on words that begin with a vowel (such as *apple*). In articulating an initial vowel sound, the larynx may first close tightly enough to build up air pressure before abruptly letting go, in order to accentuate the beginning of the sound. Because of Valsalva tuning, this original closure may turn into *effort closure,* as part of the Valsalva maneuver. You would then feel the words choking in your throat, rather than in your mouth.

Prolongation of Consonants

There are some consonants that require only a partial blockage of airflow in their articulation. These include, for example, the fricatives (*f, j, v, th, s, z, sh, zh,* and *h*), the liquids (*l* and *r*), and the semi-vowels (*w* and *y*). The air is permitted to escape through a narrowed opening between some combination of the lips, tongue, and teeth. (In the fricative *h,* the partial closure is in the false vocal cords.) Even though the blockage of airflow is not complete in these instances, it still would cause some increased air pressure in the lungs.

When Valsalva tuning occurs, the articulation of these consonants may also stimulate a Valsalva maneuver, to some extent, with closures that are more forceful than necessary. However, some of the air may continue to leak out, since the closure was never complete to begin with. The resulting sound would not only be more forced than usual, but it may be extremely prolonged. For example, you may find yourself saying, "s-s-s-s-s-salad" or "f-f-f-f-f-fries," with a continuous, prolonged hissing sound.

There are also instances when the closures are not so long or forceful, although sufficient to impede the smooth flow of speech. In these cases, the Valsalva tuning may be relatively slight. Nevertheless, *any* involvement of the Valsalva mechanism is likely to disrupt our fluency, to one degree or another.

Repetitive Stuttering

Up to this point we've talked about stuttering that consists of continuous forceful closures. This is sometimes called **tonic stuttering**, because it is similar to **tonic contractions** that occur in muscles, when they tighten in a sustained, uninterrupted way.

There is another kind of stuttering, sometimes called **clonic stuttering**, which is characterized by repetitive contractions. For example, if you were to say, "puh-puh-puh-pass the puh-puh-puh-potatoes," this might be described as clonic stuttering. It gets this name because of its similarity to **clonic spasms** that sometimes occur in muscles, when they repeatedly contract and relax in rapid succession.

Although these two types of stuttering may sound different, they actually employ the same basic mechanisms. They both involve forceful closures and increases in air pressure. The principal difference is that the first type is manifested by a single, continuous effort to force the word out, while the second is split into repeated efforts. In clonic stuttering, the person may simply come to the block, stop, and then try again, with the same result. Each time he stops, he may release air, resulting in a sound.

However, the urge to build up air pressure may be only part of the reason for the clonic type of stuttering. You might also repeat the consonant at the beginning of a word because your larynx is not ready to make the *vowel sound* that is supposed to follow.

In the next chapter, we will discuss the ways in which Valsalva tuning may interfere with phonation, resulting in various kinds of repetitive stuttering and hesitation.

Notes

See Bibliography for complete citation of references.

1. Wyke, 1971.

2. Bloodstein, 1995, p. 283; Froeschels, 1961; Soderberg, 1966; Starkweather, 1987, p. 175; Van Riper, 1982, pp. 180-181.

3. Ladefoged, 1968; Starkweather, 1987, pp. 39-44.

CHAPTER 9.

Valsalva Tuning and Phonation

THE VOICE MECHANISM of a person who stutters is often like a car with a badly tuned engine. It hesitates, it stalls, and it's hard to get started.

There may be times when we open our mouths, but nothing comes out. It seems as if our vocal cords simply won't respond to the signal to start talking. We find ourselves helplessly hesitating, because of the inability to phonate.

At other times, we may find ourselves involuntarily repeating the beginning part of a word, such as the consonant *p* in "puh-puh-puh-puh-potato." In this example, our problem may not be the consonant as much as a difficulty in moving on to the *vowel* sound that *follows* it. If our vocal cords aren't prepared to phonate at the proper time, we may get stuck on the preceding sound as we wait for the vocal cords to get ready.

As we have previously discussed, phonation is one of the basic elements of speech, together with airflow and articulation. Phonation is the vibration produced by our gently closed vocal cords as air flows between them. This vibration is shaped by our mouth and nasal cavity into the sound of our voice. Therefore, any interference with phonation is likely to disrupt the fluency of speech.

Silent Speech

If you have any doubt about the importance of phonation in stuttering, consider what happens when you talk *without phonation*. Have you ever spoken silently, without using your voice at all — simply forming the words with your mouth and letting people "read your lips"? This is sometimes called **lipped speech** or **silent articulation**.

When a stutterer uses lipped speech, without any phonation, a strange thing happens. He is able to form the words with *almost perfect fluency*.

This principle was demonstrated at a workshop I once conducted. About 28 people — all of whom stuttered — were paired off and given lists of numbered sentences. In each of the groups, one partner had to select a sentence and to mouth the words silently. The other partner tried to read his lips and guess which sentence was being read. They took turns doing this until all the sentences were completed.

When the exercise was over, I asked the participants if they had noticed any disfluency, in either themselves or their partners. To their surprise, everyone had been totally fluent during the unvoiced readings.

The same results have been achieved in scientifically controlled experiments.[1] It has been shown that *stuttering virtually disappears during silent speech*. When stutterers speak in a whisper, some disfluency may occur, but the rate is still relatively low. The full force of stuttering is not felt until the stutterer tries to speak with his voice — that is, with phonation.

Difficulties with Phonation

Why should the absence of phonation have such a dramatic impact on the elimination of stuttering?

Phonation is a complex activity involving many tiny muscles in the larynx that must move quickly and precisely. To produce a voiced sound, these muscles must bring the vocal cords together and give them just the right amount of tension to vibrate properly when airflow passes through. The tension must be adjusted during speech according to pitch, loudness, and air pressure. The vocal cords must rapidly open and close, depending on whether the sound being made is voiced or unvoiced.

Some experts have suggested that stutterers have difficulty in making these movements or in coordinating them with the various other activities of speech. When phonation is eliminated, speech becomes simpler for the stutterer to handle.[2]

Numerous studies have shown stutterers to have delays in phonation while speaking. In some of the experiments, stutterers and non-stutterers were asked to make vowel sounds in response to a signal. Invariably, the stutterers were slower.[3] Other research has discovered abnormal muscular activity in the larynx during stuttering, which may interfere with phonation.[4] Therefore, it seems clear that stutterers have difficulties and delays in phonation that play a significant role in stuttering.

These findings raise numerous questions:

Why do stutterers have problems with phonation while speaking? Why do these problems disrupt fluency *some* of the time, but not at other times? Why do stutterers become more fluent when phonation is greatly emphasized, as in *singing*? And what relationship does phonation have to other kinds of stuttering behavior, such as the forceful closures of the mouth and larynx discussed in the previous chapter?

A possible answer to all of these questions is the *neuromotor tuning of the Valsalva mechanism*, and its interference with the normal process of phonation.

Neuromotor Tuning of the Larynx

As discussed in earlier chapters, a process of neuromotor tuning takes place during the split second before normal speech, preparing the speech mechanism to perform the activities that will be required. Through this process, the brain "tunes up" the appropriate nerves and muscles of the larynx, so they will respond quickly to the triggering signals to begin phonation. At the same time, the brain normally "tunes down" other nerves and muscles — such as the Valsalva mechanism — so they will not be accidentally activated and interfere with speech.

The preparation for phonation also includes a process called **prephonatory tuning**. This adjusts the tension of the vocal cords, so they will be ready to vibrate at the right pitch as the airflow passes between them. Scientific studies have found that prephonatory tuning occurs from about one-half a second to 1/20th of a second before phonation is heard.[5]

Neuromotor and prephonatory tuning continue throughout normal speech. As we are making one sound, our nervous system is already preparing our speech mechanism to make the sound that follows it. If everything is tuned properly, one sound should flow smoothly into the next, without interruption. On the other hand, if something interferes with the tuning of a stutterer's larynx, the result could be delays in phonation, hesitations, repetitions, and other stuttering behavior.

The Valsalva Hypothesis offers a logical explanation of how this interference might happen. In times of stress, when we anticipate that speaking will be difficult, our brain may neurologically "tune up" our body's Valsalva mechanism, preparing it to "force" the words out by means of a Valsalva maneuver. The larynx, as we know, is an important part of the Valsalva mechanism. Therefore, any tuning of the Valsalva mechanism is likely to affect the larynx.

If the larynx is tuned for a Valsalva maneuver, it is *not* ready for phonation. It is not ready to bring the vocal cords gently together, with the proper tension to vibrate as airflow passes between them. Instead, the larynx is ready to perform *effort closure* — an entirely different function, in which both the vocal cords and false cords squeeze shut, in order to prevent air from leaving the lungs.

Even if our larynx does not actually close, our vocal cords are not ready to vibrate at the proper time. Therefore, when the triggering signal comes for the voice to kick in, nothing happens. This delay in phonation will interfere with the flow of speech, as we struggle to re-tune the larynx to make the proper sound.

In some cases, our struggle to phonate may only make the problem worse. When our voice fails to respond on cue, this may confirm our fears that speech will be difficult and that extra effort is needed. In response, our brain may send additional signals to tune up the Valsalva mechanism.

The more we tune up the Valsalva mechanism,

the less we are ready to phonate. And the less we are ready to phonate, the more we may tune up the Valsalva mechanism, in a misguided attempt to force the word out. The result is a vicious cycle that further delays phonation.

Force and Phonation

The Valsalva mechanism's sole purpose is to build up air pressure in the lungs, thereby enabling us to exert physical effort more efficiently. The air pressure is increased by tightening the chest and abdominal muscles, while forcefully closing the mouth or larynx to keep the air from escaping. Therefore, the further tuning of the Valsalva mechanism would not only prolong our hesitations and repetitions by delaying phonation, but could also cause *forceful closures of our mouth and larynx*, as discussed in the previous chapter.

From personal experience, I have found that stuttering is usually a *combination* of the difficulty to phonate and the use of excessive force. When I had trouble in voicing a sound, I would feel an overwhelming urge to build up air pressure in an attempt to force the sound out. This would be done by closing my mouth or larynx, while contracting my chest and abdominal muscles, as in a Valsalva maneuver.

I seemed to forget that there is only one way to phonate — to bring the vocal cords gently together across a flow of air. Instead, I found myself using force and air pressure as if they were a *substitute* for phonation. The force and air pressure made me *feel* as if I were doing something that might help to get the word out. But, in reality, it was useless. This kind of behavior could not possibly give voice to my speech. On the contrary, it produced forceful closures of the mouth or larynx that blocked my speech more than ever.

Effect of Phonation on Fluency

The Valsalva Hypothesis ties together the two principal characteristics of stuttering — excessive force and delays in phonation. It can also explain why we become more fluent when we *emphasize phonation* — for example, when we *sing*.

Most stutterers are totally fluent while singing.[6] If we compare singing to ordinary speech, we find that the biggest difference is in the way we phonate. During singing, we rely on phonation to carry the melody. We stretch out the vowels. We phonate almost all the time.[7]

When we sing, our mind concentrates on the melody, rather than worrying about how to force the words out. Therefore, our neuromotor tuning is focused on *phonation*, rather than on a Valsalva maneuver. Our brain is busy sending signals to the larynx to adjust the pitch of our vocal cords and to modulate the tone of our voice. Consequently, our larynx is always ready to phonate at the proper time.

"Tuning up" the larynx for phonation also has the effect of "tuning down" the Valsalva mechanism throughout the entire body. Relaxing one part of the Valsalva mechanism has a tendency to relax the other parts as well. The urge to build up air pressure is reduced. There is less chance that the mouth or larynx will close forcefully to block the airflow. As a result, our stuttering disappears.

As we shall discuss in subsequent chapters, there are many other circumstances that improve fluency by emphasizing phonation. Some techniques — such as talking with slow speech or stretched syllables — increase phonation by prolonging the vowel sounds. Other forms of therapy teach the stutterer to keep his larynx constantly phonating or ready to phonate. These methods come under various labels, including "continuous phonation," "legato speech," and "vocal control therapy," and also play a role in a number of "fluency shaping" programs. Technology has also gotten into the act, in the form of electronic gadgets that help the stutterer to monitor the vibration of his larynx.

To the extent that these methods are successful, the reason is the same. By focusing the stutterer's attention on phonation, they improve the neuromotor and prephonatory tuning of the larynx. This enables the larynx to phonate more readily, relaxes the Valsalva mechanism, and reduces the likelihood of a Valsalva maneuver.

Now that we have established the principles behind the two basic manifestations of stuttering — forceful closures and difficulty in phonation — we are ready to analyze and understand a wide array of stuttering and avoidance behaviors.

✧

Notes

See Bibliography for complete citations of references.

1. Perkins, Rudas, and Johnson, 1976.

2. Perkins, Rudas, and Johnson, 1976.

3. Adams and Reis, 1971; Adams, 1974; Bakker and Brutten, 1989, 1990; Borden, Baer, and Kenney, 1985; Healey and Gutkin, 1984; Mallard, Hicks, and Riggs, 1982; Reich, Till, And Goldsmith, 1981; Starkweather, Hirschman and Tannenbaum, 1976; Starkweather, Franklin, and Smigo, 1984; Starkweather, 1987, pp. 235-243.

4. Conture, McCall, and Brewer, 1977; Conture, Schwartz, and Brewer, 1985; Freeman, Ushijima, and Hirose, 1975; Shapiro, 1980.

5. Wyke, 1971.

6. Bloodstein, 1995, pp. 297, 304; Starkweather, 1987, p. 190; Van Riper, 1982, p. 425; Wingate, 1969.

7. Wingate, 1969.

Part IV.

Perpetuation of Stuttering Behavior

CHAPTER 10.

Varieties of Stuttering

IMAGINE THAT YOU ARE HIKING down a country road. Suddenly you come upon a high stone wall with a big, solid gate closed across your path. You push against the gate, but it won't open. You push harder, you pound repeatedly, but still it won't budge.

Other travelers arrive. They also push and pound on the gate, to no avail. Then each individual comes up with a different method of attacking the problem. One takes a running start and throws his whole body against the gate. Another finds a crowbar and tries to pry the gate open. Others attempt to climb over the wall.

Some travelers wander off the road, in search of a route around the wall. Still others, having learned that there is a gatekeeper on the other side, use various ploys to trick him into opening the gate. They will wait for the gate to open and then try to dash through before it shuts again.

This story illustrates how a single obstacle — the closed gate — can provoke a wide variety of responses. The actions of the individual travelers may be different, but the underlying obstacle is the same. None of the pushing, pounding, running, climbing, and other strategies would have been necessary if the travelers simply had a key to open the gate.

Those of us who stutter may find ourselves in a similar situation. For us, the road is speech. The closed gate is the blockage of speech. When we experience or anticipate this obstacle, we may find ourselves doing a wide assortment of puzzling things.

These behaviors go beyond the forceful closures and difficulties in phonation discussed in the previous chapters. A few of the more common examples are:
- Hesitations;
- Repetitions of sounds, words, phrases, and even whole sentences;
- The use of "uh's," "ah's," stock phrases (e.g., "you know," "let's see"), and other unnecessary words and sounds;
- Word substitutions and circumlocutions;
- Grunting, gasping, panting, and other breathing irregularities;
- Facial contortions, teeth gnashing, arm swinging, and other bodily movements.

There is almost no limit to the bizarre things we might do in our struggle to speak. However, the superficial differences do not mean that each behavior has a cause that is separate and distinct from other types of stuttering. Like the travelers' activities in the story, *the various stuttering behaviors may all be attempts to overcome or avoid the same underlying obstacle.* I myself have, at one time or another, engaged in almost every variety of stuttering that I have ever seen.

In order to understand how these behaviors fit into the overall stuttering picture, we must first distinguish between the underlying obstacle to speech (the closed gate) and those activities that are in response to the obstacle.

Direct and Indirect Symptoms

In the previous chapters, we have identified

Chapter 10 / Varieties of Stuttering

two basic manifestations of stuttering: (1) excessively forceful closures of the mouth or larynx, and (2) difficulty in phonation. We will refer to these as the **direct symptoms** of stuttering.

We have seen how both of these aspects of stuttering can be explained by the *neuromotor tuning of the Valsalva mechanism*. Such tuning is most likely to occur when we anticipate that speaking will be difficult and we feel the need to use extra effort to force the words out.

As a result, the muscles of our larynx, mouth, chest, and abdomen become ready to perform a *Valsalva maneuver* — an instinctive bodily function that ordinarily helps us to exert strenuous physical effort or to force things out of our abdomen (such as a bowel movement). The Valsalva maneuver is done by forcefully closing the upper airway at the larynx or mouth, while contracting the chest and abdominal muscles to build up air pressure in the lungs. As air pressure builds up, the larynx or mouth automatically closes more tightly to keep the air from escaping. Therefore, the harder we force, the more our speech is blocked by the closure.

We have also seen that, when our larynx is neurologically tuned for a Valsalva maneuver, it is *not* ready to produce the phonation necessary for the sound of our voice. The resulting delay in phonation can interrupt our speech, even without a closure of our mouth or larynx.

These two aspects of stuttering may work in combination with one another. When phonation fails, there may be an urge to build up air pressure in an attempt to force the sound out. However, this only leads to forceful closures of the mouth or larynx and a greater blockage of speech.

Therefore, either or both of these two aspects of stuttering may cause the underlying blockage of speech. Each individual might then react to this obstacle in different ways, in an attempt either (1) to break through a stuttering block as it is encountered, or (2) to avoid, postpone, or conceal a block that is anticipated.

The result may be a wide variety of struggle and avoidance behaviors, which become a habitual part of the individual's own pattern of stuttering. We will refer to these behaviors as the **indirect symptoms** of stuttering.

Now let's examine a number of these behaviors to see how they might have come about.

Hesitations

Hesitations in speech may be a direct result of the forceful closures and difficulties in phonation previously described. If airflow is blocked or phonation is disrupted, there will inevitably be an interruption in speech — and therefore hesitation.

We may also hesitate when we *anticipate* that a block is coming. Rather than crashing into the block head on, we might simply wait for the pressure to subside. If we can't find our voice, we might pause until our larynx gets ready to phonate. If we are patient enough, the block may eventually go away.

Waiting out a stuttering block might sound simple, but it can be murder during an actual conversation. Silence is extremely uncomfortable, both to the speaker and the listener. If we pause too long, the other person might either: (a) interrupt us by starting to talk; or (b) lose interest, walk away, or hang up the phone. Therefore, we may feel ourselves under great social pressure to show the other person that we are still trying to communicate. Doing or saying *something*, almost *anything*, may feel preferable to remaining silent.

The fear of silence is an important motivation for many kinds of stuttering behavior. Most of us will not simply stop, relax, and wait for a block to pass. Instead, we may either: (1) show that we are struggling to talk, or (2) say something else that we feel won't be blocked.

Signs of Struggle

There are many ways to show the listener that we haven't quit speaking, but are struggling to break through a block. If we really want to show how hard we are trying, we can go into a full-blown Valsalva maneuver, squeezing our mouth or larynx closed as we build up air pressure, perhaps until we are red in the face.

Or we may split the Valsalva maneuver into a series of short bursts of effort. At the end of each burst, the mouth or larynx opens, releasing an audible sound. When the struggle is in the mouth, the resulting sound may be a repetition of the beginning of a word. ("P-p-p-p-pass the p-p-p-p-potatoes.") When the struggle is in the larynx, the result may be a series of little grunts ("Uh-uh-uh-

uh-uh").

Other muscles may be brought into the struggle. Facial contortions may occur as we strain various muscles in an attempt to pull the mouth open. Or we may try to pry the mouth open by shifting the pressure onto the jaw instead. However, the forceful closure of the jaw only results in a painful clenching and gnashing of the teeth, sometimes causing us to bite the inside of our mouth.

This struggle can expand even beyond the mouth and face, as more and more parts of the body become involved. We may end up with eyes closing, neck jerking, arms swinging, fists clenching, feet stomping, and so on.

Starters, Fillers, and Other Junk Words

Another way to fill in the silence is to say things that are not likely to cause us to block. The most common examples are **starters** and **fillers**. These include meaningless sounds like "uh" and "ah," and stock phrases like "you know" and "let's see." Although normal speakers occasionally use these verbal crutches, stutterers are world champions at this activity. ("Uh, well, would you pass, you know, like, pass the, let's see, uh, the potatoes?")

Because these are "junk" words — with no value or meaning — we feel no need to "try hard" to say them properly. Therefore, neuromotor tuning of the Valsalva mechanism is less likely to occur and we are less likely to block. Unfortunately, we may overuse them to such a degree that they become more annoying than either stuttering or silence would have been.

This might also explain why it was easier for me to say the wrong thing rather than the precise thing I wanted to say.

The stutterer may also fill in the silence by repeating what has already been said. This may be a word, phrase, or entire sentence. Having already been said, it is no longer important. Therefore, there will be less of an urge to try hard to say it, and the Valsalva mechanism will be less likely to interfere.

There is a common misconception that the repeated word is the one on which we are blocking. On the contrary, we are repeating it precisely because it is *not* giving us trouble. Usually we are anticipating a block on the word that *follows* it.

In addition to filling in the silence, starters and repetitions may be used as a "running start" in attacking a word we fear will be difficult. Whether this really helps is questionable. Often I hear stutterers repeating whole sentences, over and over, only to stop abruptly when they reach the feared word. The effect on the listener can be maddening.

Word Substitution

When we find ourselves blocking on a particular word, we may attempt to avoid the block by substituting another word in its place. A substitute word is usually easier to say, because it is not what we had really *wanted* to say.

Again, the reason may lie in Valsalva tuning. All our effort was focused on properly saying the precise word that we had chosen. This caused the Valsalva mechanism to be activated, resulting in a block. Since the substitute word has less importance to us, we feel no need to use extra effort to say it. Therefore, the Valsalva mechanism doesn't get involved and we can say the substitute word more fluently.

Word substitution can be carried to such an extreme that it becomes **circumlocution**. That is, a person may rephrase entire sentences in an effort to avoid stuttering on certain words. "Please pass the potatoes" may thus be transformed into "Kindly send over that bowl of mashed-up stuff." The stutterer tries to sustain an illusion of fluency by sacrificing the right to say what he really wants.

Timing Irregularities

A stutterer's speech is rarely smooth. It often proceeds in a jerky fashion, at one moment lurching ahead with a rapid burst of words, then grinding to a halt. This tendency has led some experts to suspect that stuttering is caused by a lack of timing and coordination. However, it is also possible that jerky speech is a habit developed in an attempt to "fake out" the stuttering block.

We may race through the words, hoping to outrun the block before it catches up with us. Or we may try to sneak up on the block, and then rush through. We change rhythm or verbally bob and weave like basketball players, as ploys to catch

Chapter 10 / Varieties of Stuttering

the block off guard.

Breathing Irregularities

Persons who stutter may also do puzzling things with their breathing. These include huffing, puffing, panting, snorting, gasping, trying to speak with little or no air in the lungs, and trying to speak while inhaling. We don't do these things intentionally. They just seem to happen sometimes, when we feel a block coming on.

For example, I once had a tendency to huff and puff before answering the telephone. Upon closer examination, I found that I was rapidly contracting my chest and abdominal muscles, in response to an overwhelming urge to build up air pressure. Even though my mouth and larynx were open, these rapid contractions still resulted in temporary increases of air pressure in the lungs. I wasn't doing a full Valsalva maneuver, because my upper airway wasn't closed. Nevertheless, this behavior indicated that at least part of the Valsalva mechanism was at work.

At other times, I noticed a great struggle going on between the muscles of the chest and abdomen. It seemed as if the muscles for inhaling were straining to keep the chest expanded, while the muscles of the Valsalva mechanism were squeezing to compress the chest cavity. The two opposing forces seemed to have reached a stalemate, so the air pressure in the lungs did not increase. My mouth and larynx remained open, but no air was moving in or out.

Again, I had the impression that at least part of the Valsalva mechanism was at work. It felt as if the Valsalva mechanism was trying to exert force through the muscles of the abdomen and the chest muscles that are used to force air out, but was thwarted by opposing sets of muscles. Although the Valsalva maneuver had been defeated, the victory was meaningless, since there was no airflow for speech.

Trying to speak without air in the lungs may be another attempt to head off a Valsalva maneuver. Obviously, we can't build up much air pressure in the lungs if we don't have much air to start with. But this practice also interferes with speech by depriving us of airflow.

Habits of Desperation

This discussion has touched on only some of the behaviors that stutterers adopt in their effort to overcome or avoid stuttering blocks.

Most of the strategies are stumbled upon in desperation, usually without conscious thought. At first they may seem better than nothing, even though they disrupt speech in ways of their own. And so we return to them, again and again. Eventually, they become a habitual part of our individual pattern of stuttering. These behaviors may become as deeply entrenched, and as much of a problem, as the primary stuttering blocks that they were intended to combat.

In the next chapter, we will observe how stuttering behavior, our negative reactions to our speech, and the Valsalva mechanism may all reinforce one another, drawing us into a vicious circle.

General References

BLOODSTEIN, O. *A Handbook on Stuttering.* 5th ed. San Diego: Singular Publishing Group, 1995, pp. 11-22.
STARKWEATHER, C. W. *Fluency and Stuttering.* Englewood Cliffs, N.J.: Prentice-Hall, 1987, pp. 117-127.
VAN RIPER, C. *The Nature of Stuttering.* 2nd ed. Englewood Cliffs, N.J.: Prentice-Hall, 1982, pp. 111-143.

CHAPTER 11.

The Valsalva-Stuttering Cycle

THE CIRCLE is a fundamental pattern found throughout nature. It is not merely a shape. It is a system in which one event leads to another, eventually arriving at the starting point, where the same events are repeated again and again, in a continuing cycle.

Examples are everywhere: the alternation of day and night, the changing seasons, water evaporating into the air and falling as rain, the reproductive cycles of living things. Human beings have incorporated the circle into countless inventions, beginning with the wheel.

The beauty of the circle is that it has no fixed beginning or end. Therefore, it can repeat itself indefinitely. Unfortunately, this same pattern on which life depends can also serve to perpetuate undesirable results. When this happens, it is sometimes called a **vicious circle**.

Stuttering also follows a circular pattern, which neither begins nor ends with the disfluency itself. The physical aspects of stuttering, described in the previous chapters, are preceded and followed by psychological expectations and reactions. These mental factors interact with the physical factors, including the Valsalva mechanism, to create a vicious circle, which both stimulates and perpetuates our stuttering behavior. We shall call this the **Valsalva-Stuttering Cycle**.

The Valsalva-Stuttering cycle has the following major elements:

(a) Psychological and emotional factors, such as our negative feelings about speech and our expectation of difficulty;

(b) Our neurological response to those feelings, in terms of neuromotor tuning of the Valsalva mechanism;

(c) The physical effects of Valsalva tuning, which interfere with speech;

(d) Various behaviors we adopt in an attempt to break through or avoid the blocks; and

(e) Our mental reactions to our stuttering, which confirm and strengthen our negative feelings and expectations about speech, bringing us back to point (a).

We will now travel through the Valsalva-Stuttering cycle (which is graphically depicted in the accompanying diagram) and follow the sequence of events in greater detail.

Step 1. The Anticipation of Difficulty. Let us begin our description of the Valsalva-Stuttering cycle by considering the mental attitudes we bring into a speaking situation. As we have seen, we tend to stutter more when we feel that the words themselves are especially important, or we anticipate that speaking will be difficult.

Often we expect difficulty in saying a particular word or sound. One week we may have problems with the letter *p*. The next week it may be the letter *f*. The words or sounds that bother us are based on our own personal experiences and feelings. If we have had trouble with them in the past, we expect trouble in the future.

The same is true with specific speaking situations. Some people may expect more difficulty when using the telephone, or when talking to authority figures, such as parents, teachers, bosses, policemen, judges, or other people they feel they have to please or impress. The fear becomes particularly great when we try to hide the fact that we stutter.

The anticipation of difficulty may also be influenced by ambivalence, uncertainty, emotional conflict, and a variety of other psychological factors, to be discussed in the next chapter. Among these is the self-image we may have of ourselves as stutterers. It might also be aggravated, in some instances, by the stutterer's feeling of having an impaired speaking ability due to fatigue, illness, inexperience, or other factors. As we shall discuss in subsequent chapters, some individuals may also have neurological weaknesses that increase the difficulty of speech to varying degrees.

We may have become so accustomed to these mental attitudes that we no longer give them any conscious thought. Nevertheless, they set in motion a chain of events that lead to stuttering.

Step 2. The Urge To "Try Hard." Because we expect difficulty in speaking, it is natural for us to feel that extra effort may be needed to get us over the hurdles. However, we may forget the fact that speech is simply phonation and a sequence of movements. We may forget that fluent speech requires very little physical effort, and that force can only interfere.

Instead, we may have a tendency to treat words as if they were "things" that can be forced out by physical effort. For some reason, we cling to the idea that we can help our speech by using the same kind of physical force that is normally assisted by the body's Valsalva mechanism. The result may be an urge to "try hard" in a physical way.

Step 3. Valsalva Tuning. The brain responds to our urge to try hard by sending nerve impulses to the larynx and other parts of the body's Valsalva mechanism, preparing them to exert physical force by means of a Valsalva maneuver. This preparation is done by the process of neuromotor tuning, previously discussed.

As we have seen, a Valsalva maneuver is a normal bodily function that is designed to assist us in exerting physical effort and in forcing things out of the abdomen. It is done by forcefully closing the upper airway at the larynx or mouth, while contracting the chest and abdominal muscles to build up air pressure in the lungs.

During a Valsalva maneuver, the larynx normally performs a function known as effort closure, in which it closes tightly to prevent air from leaving the lungs.

Step 4. Vocal Delays and Forceful Closures. Because of Valsalva tuning, the larynx is neurologically prepared for the exertion of force, rather than phonation. Even if it does not actually close tightly, the larynx is not ready to produce the vocal sounds at the precise times when they are needed for speech. The interference with phonation may confirm our fears that speech will indeed be difficult. This increases our urge to try hard to force the words out.

Valsalva tuning also increases the likelihood that the mouth or larynx will instinctively close with excessive force during articulation. We have referred to these two symptoms — *difficulty in phonation* and *excessively forceful closures* — as the **direct symptoms** of stuttering.

Step 5. Avoidance Behavior. In an attempt to avoid, postpone, or hide the blocks caused by the vocal delays and forceful closures, we may resort to various kinds of behavior, described in the previous chapter. A few examples are hesitations, repetitions, the use of starters, fillers, and other unnecessary words and sounds, word substitutions and circumlocutions, grunting, gasping, and other breathing irregularities, timing irregularities, facial contortions, teeth gnashing, and other bodily movements.

Step 6. Mental Reaction to Stuttering. After the stuttering episode is over, the next part of the cycle is the way that we *mentally react* to our experience. If we had a hard struggle trying to get the words out, there is a natural tendency for us to confirm our worst expectations about the difficulty of speech.

We may think, "I was right. That *was* difficult. If I didn't try hard, I probably *never* would have been able to say it. The next time I'll have to try even *harder*."

When finally the block dissipates and the word comes out, our struggle seems to be rewarded. We are left with the false impression that the Valsalva tuning, the use of force, and other stuttering behaviors were actually successful in overcoming the obstacle. Ironically, the same behaviors that *created* the stuttering are given credit for rescuing us from the difficulty. Although the stuttering itself was miserable, we are grateful that at least we survived the ordeal. As a result, *we tend to reinforce the very activities that will promote stuttering in the future.*

THE VALSALVA-STUTTERING CYCLE

1. Anticipation of Difficulty
Expectation that speaking will be difficult, or that a particular word or sound will be hard to say. Concern over importance of good speech. Fear, emotional conflict, or ambivalence about talking. Fear of stuttering. Feeling of impaired speaking ability due to fatigue, illness, inexperience, neurological deficits, etc. Self-image as a stutterer.

2. Urge To "Try Hard"
The feeling that physical effort will be needed to force the words out and to overcome the obstacles to speech. The person may unconsciously treat the words as if they were "things" that can be forced out with the same kind of physical effort that is normally assisted by the body's Valsalva mechanism.

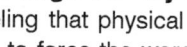

3. Valsalva Tuning
The brain responds by neurologically preparing the larynx and other parts of the body's Valsalva mechanism to perform a Valsalva maneuver (in which air pressure is built up by forcefully closing the larynx or mouth while the chest and abdominal muscles squeeze the chest cavity), in the mistaken belief that this may help to force the words out.

4. Vocal Delays and Forceful Closures
Difficulty or delays in phonation, because the larynx is neurologically prepared to perform effort closure rather than phonation. Valsalva tuning also leads to excessively forceful closures of the mouth or larynx during articulation, resulting in the blockage of speech.

5. Avoidance Behaviors
Attempts to overcome, avoid, postpone, or hide the blockage of speech. May involve a wide variety of behaviors, such as hesitations, repetitions, use of starters, fillers, and other unnecessary words and sounds, word substitutions, grunting, breathing irregularities, facial contortions, teeth gnashing, etc.

6. Mental Reaction
Confirmation of belief that speaking is difficult, or that a particular word or sound is hard to say. False impression that force or other stuttering behavior helped to get the words out. Reinforcement of Valsalva tuning, the use of force, and stuttering behavior as ways of overcoming obstacles. Feelings of guilt, shame, and embarrassment. Loss of confidence and self-esteem.

Our evaluation of our speech also may reinforce negative ideas and feeling about ourselves. We may lose confidence in our ability to talk. We may feel embarrassed, ashamed, and guilty. For some people, the result can be a tremendous loss of self-esteem.

The next time a speaking situation comes around, we may have increasingly negative expectations. Because speech was difficult the previous time, we anticipate that it will be difficult again. This may provoke an urge to try even harder than before, which may stimulate even greater Valsalva tuning and even more severe blocking.

The Valsalva-Stuttering cycle may turn from a vicious circle into a **vicious spiral.** When we are in a downward spiral, we not only go round and round, but every time we complete the circle, we find ourselves at a point lower than before. Our rut becomes ever deeper and harder to escape. We are caught in the "Valsalva Trap."

Variations and Sub-Cycles. Thus far, we have described a basic cycle, covering one stuttering episode to the next. To this may be added many variations, depending on the individual and the situation. Sometimes there may be smaller sub-cycles, in which certain steps are bypassed. For example, in some instances, the avoidance behavior (Step 5) may be skipped. In others, the anticipation of difficulty may lead *directly into* avoidance behavior.

Our speech may also be subject to ups and downs that seem to follow larger cyclical patterns as well. For days or weeks we may enjoy relative fluency, only to slip suddenly into a period of severe stuttering.

The question of whether we will stutter, under what circumstances, and how severely cannot be determined by physical factors alone. Each individual's stuttering is influenced by a lifetime accumulation of emotional baggage, which can make it as unique as his or her personality. In the next chapter, we shall examine some of the psychological and emotional factors that may affect stuttering.

CHAPTER 12.

The Psychology of Stuttering

NO DESCRIPTION of stuttering is complete without accounting for the great variability we see in stuttering behavior — not only between different stutterers, but even within the same individual. My own experience is a good example.

Back when I stuttered severely, I often couldn't say a fluent sentence in a one-to-one conversation. However, I could stand before a large audience and act out a role with perfect fluency. I could also be quite fluent when making an impassioned argument, or when letting out my anger at someone. At one time, I was both the best and worst speaker in my high school class.

Such variables have, in the past, led some experts to conclude that stuttering was a purely **psychoneurotic disorder**, caused by emotional conflicts or other traumatic events that were repressed into the unconscious mind. This was, in fact, the prevailing view of stuttering from the early twentieth century through the 1960's.

Many psychiatrists attempted to explain stuttering solely in Freudian psychoanalytic terms, rejecting any possibility of physiological factors. According to some theories, stuttering was due to an **oral fixation**, in which the stutterer unconsciously desired to suck or bite as if he were nursing. Others saw stuttering in terms of an **anal fixation**, reflecting the stutterer's conflict over expelling or retaining words as if they were feces. Still other theories viewed stuttering as an **ego-defect neurosis** involving certain kinds of conflict, anxiety, and ambivalence engendered by the stutterer's mother.

These theories were of little practical value in the treatment of stuttering. Even worse, they did considerable damage by causing stuttering to be lumped into the category of "mental illness," thereby subjecting stutterers to untold prejudice and misunderstanding. Furthermore, they were contradicted by studies that showed stutterers, as a group, to be no more neurotic or emotionally disturbed than the general population.

In reaction to the psychoanalytic theories, some experts completely rejected the importance of emotional factors in stuttering. They tried to explain stuttering solely in terms of either (a) learned or conditioned behavior, or (b) physical or neurological defects. It became popular to treat stuttering by various means of behavior modification, on a purely mechanical level. However, these approaches were also incomplete. They failed to explain or resolve the psychological and emotional obstacles to fluency, which usually returned soon after the stutterer left the therapist's office.

Psychological Factors

The inescapable conclusion — already mentioned in our previous chapters — is that stuttering arises from the interplay of *both* physical *and* psychological factors. According to the Valsalva hypothesis, the speech mechanism of a person who stutters has the basic capability of fluent speech. Under certain circumstances, however, the person's larynx and other muscles become neurologically tuned for a Valsalva maneuver, which may interfere with phonation and speech. The degree of such tuning might be influenced by psychological and emotional factors, and would more likely occur in those instances when the person feels a

Chapter 12 / The Psychology of Stuttering

particular need to "try hard" to get the words out.

In the previous chapter, we saw how both psychological and physical factors work together, in a vicious circle, to promote and perpetuate stuttering. The basic *psychological* elements of the Valsalva-Stuttering Cycle are:

• Our anticipation, belief, or feeling that speaking will be difficult (Step 1);

• Our urge to use physical effort to force out the words (Step 2), which leads to the activation of the Valsalva mechanism and stuttering; and

• Our mental evaluation or perception of the stuttering experience, which reinforces our belief that speech is difficult and that force is needed to overcome the obstacle (Step 6).

As we have seen, our primary negative belief is that *speech is a difficult task that requires physical effort to force the words out.* This negative anticipation may be increased in regard to specific words, sounds, or speaking situations that we believe will be particularly difficult (perhaps due to our past experiences).

Our anticipation of difficulty then triggers an urge to "try hard" or to use physical effort to overcome the anticipated obstacle to speech. This urge then interacts with the physical side of the circle, by causing the neurological tuning of the body's Valsalva mechanism, leading to stuttering.

The psychological side of the circle then resumes with our mental reaction to the stuttering experience. These perceptions may confirm our belief that speech is difficult and that perhaps even *greater* force will be needed in the future.

Learning and Conditioning

To some extent, the perpetuation and entrenchment of the stuttering cycle might be explained in terms of **learned** or **conditioned behavior**. It is well known that certain behaviors can be established by a psychological process called **conditioning** — sometimes referred to as "the carrot and the stick" principle.

The basic concept is simple. When a person's behavior is followed by a reward (usually something pleasurable), he will tend to repeat the same behavior in the future. Such a reward is called **positive reinforcement**. On the other hand, if a particular behavior is followed by a punishment (called **negative reinforcement**), he will tend to avoid that behavior.

Beginning in early childhood, we learn numerous behavior patterns through the everyday operation of conditioning. However, the process sometimes leads to unexpected results, because some kinds of behavior produce both rewards *and* punishments. Stuttering is a prime example.

On the surface, stuttering behavior might be viewed as pure punishment. Stuttering is inherently unpleasant, and it sometimes provokes adverse responses (such as ridicule) from other people. Why, then, don't these negative reinforcements stop us from stuttering?

The reason is that, on another level, the stuttering behavior is being strengthened by *positive* reinforcement. Remember, we entered the speaking situation with the belief that speech would be difficult. We responded to that belief by activating our Valsalva mechanism, in order to "try hard" to force the words out. After the struggle is over, and the words finally get out, our *perception* is that *the obstacle has been overcome*, and that *the use of force was successful in doing so*. Although the stuttering itself was a punishing experience, we are relieved that it's over. In this way, *the use of force is rewarded*.

The combined result of these negative and positive reinforcements is doubly damaging. The negative reinforcement of stuttering teaches us to fear speaking situations and to try to hide our stuttering. This strengthens our belief that speaking will be difficult and will require extra effort. The positive reinforcement of force teaches us to activate our Valsalva mechanism and to use excessive force while speaking. Ironically, *our minds tend to view Valsalva tuning and force as our saviors, rather than the culprits they really are!*

Individual Variations

The basic stuttering cycle is subject to infinite variations, depending on the unique personality and psychological make-up of each individual. In particular, we all have somewhat different anticipations about the difficulty of speech, based on our own individual histories. As a general rule, we are more likely to anticipate difficulty with respect to those words, situations, and listeners that seemed to cause stuttering in the past. Conversely, we will tend to anticipate *less* difficulty with respect to situations that have seemed easy and pleasant in the past.

Our anticipation of difficulty might be further stirred up by any number of things that remind us of previous stuttering experiences. For example, it could be the ringing of the telephone, some aspect of the listener's appearance or manner, the topic being discussed, or significant details about the surroundings. These and other factors that stimulate the anticipation of stuttering are sometimes called **cues**. Although we are not always conscious of them, they may affect our speech to a greater extent than we ever realize.

Another important factor is the *image we have of ourselves as speakers*. The very fact that a person believes that he is a "stutterer" may carry with it the anticipation that speech will be difficult. If the person also feels that stuttering is shameful and should be hidden, his urge to use excessive effort in speaking may be further compounded. Unfortunately, it is not always easy to change these beliefs. A person's self-image as a stutterer may become such a fundamental part of his personality that he cannot abandon it without suffering a terrible sense of anxiety or loss. Such feelings can sabotage any attempts at stuttering therapy.

Emotional Conflict

Even if we don't buy any of the psychoanalytic theories, we can't rule out *emotion* as a possible factor in stuttering behavior. Emotional conflict, uncertainty, and ambivalence may naturally interfere with anybody's speech. These feelings may be stirred up by various speaking situations, for reasons that are personal to each individual. Like the other psychological factors, they may also be unconscious.

For the stutterer, emotional conflicts can be particularly troublesome, because they may further increase the anticipation that speech will be difficult. Therefore, emotional conflicts may serve as a trigger for stuttering. In addition, the struggle of stuttering may serve as a battleground on which the conflicts are then acted out.

Through speech, we communicate more than just words. We reach out and touch people with our feelings. However, if we feel so conflicted that we can't express these feelings, we may end up holding back our words also. Consequently, we may find ourselves in an **approach-avoidance conflict** in which, on the one hand, we want to express ourselves, but on the other, we are afraid to do so.

We may use the Valsalva maneuver as a means of acting out this ambivalence. It is perfectly designed for such a struggle, because it involves two conflicting forces: a physical effort to force air outward, while at the same time an equally forceful effort to hold the air in.

In my own case, stuttering was worst when I felt tied up in emotional knots, when I felt confused, conflicted, and uncertain. In contrast, when my emotions all were in harmony and aimed in the same direction, my speech just seemed to flow along with the current. In those cases, I felt less of a need to use extra effort. Therefore, the Valsalva mechanism stayed relaxed, and speech came with less effort and greater fluency.

Secondary Benefits of Stuttering

Stuttering is not something that we would consciously choose to do. However, after having been stuck with it for a while, we may have learned ways to turn it to our advantage. As a result, we may be reaping **secondary benefits** from stuttering that serve to reinforce our continued stuttering behavior.

To some people, stuttering becomes a refuge, a convenient excuse for not doing things, not meeting people, not talking on the phone, not subjecting oneself to fearful situations. It can be a rationalization for not taking control over our lives, or for not having achieved all the great things we might have.

Through stuttering, we might avoid the fear of expressing ourselves or taking responsibility for our words and thoughts. I myself once fell into this habit. If I had a conflict over what to say, I would just open my mouth and start stuttering. I figured that there was no sense in choosing my words carefully if I wasn't going to be able to say them anyway.

Stuttering may also be used as a display of great effort, calculated to gain pity or indulgence (especially if the listener is an authority figure of some kind). By doing a Valsalva maneuver, or by struggling over our words, we are showing the listener *how hard we are trying to talk.* The unconscious message might be: "You can't punish me. It's not *my* fault that I stutter. Look how *hard* I'm trying to please you!"

Although this tactic may seem rather childish, as viewed by an adult stutterer, we must remember that stuttering almost always *begins in childhood.* Many of us learned as children that "trying hard" is supposed to be *good*. If we can't do well, at least we can get an "A" for effort.

Furthermore, the Valsalva maneuver is a universal way of expressing effort. When a child makes a grunting sound, to show that he is straining hard, he is audibly demonstrating a Valsalva maneuver.

In the next chapter, we will further explore the origins of stuttering in childhood, and demonstrate how simple disfluencies can develop into struggle behavior and chronic stuttering.

General References

BLOODSTEIN, O. *A Handbook on Stuttering.* 5th ed. San Diego: Singular Publishing Group, 1995, pp. 61-66, 211-237.

FREUND, H. *Psychopathology and the Problems of Stuttering.* Springfield, Ill.: Charles C. Thomas, 1966.

GLAUBER, I. P. Dynamic therapy for the stutterer. *Specialized Techniques in Psychotherapy.* New York: Grove Press, 1952, 207-238.

SHEEHAN, J. G. Theory and treatment of stuttering as an approach-avoidance conflict. *Stuttering Then and Now* (edited by Shames, G.H., & Rubin, H.). Columbus, OH: Charles E. Merrill Publishing Co., 1986, 187-200.

TRAVIS, L. E. The unspeakable feelings of people with special reference to stuttering. Emotional factors. *Stuttering Then and Now* (edited by Shames, G.H., & Rubin, H.). Columbus, OH: Charles E. Merrill Publishing Co., 1986, 93-122.

VAN RIPER, C. *The Nature of Stuttering.* 2nd ed. Englewood Cliffs, N.J.: Prentice-Hall, 1982, pp. 261-322.

Part V.

Susceptibility to Stuttering

CHAPTER 13.

The Origins of Stuttering

IN PREVIOUS CHAPTERS, we have viewed stuttering in its fully developed, chronic form. We have seen how our body's Valsalva mechanism might be activated when we anticipate trouble speaking, resulting in delayed phonation and stuttering blocks. We have seen how a combination of physical and psychological factors might reinforce one another to create the Valsalva-Stuttering Cycle that perpetuates this behavior.

These are the factors we must understand if we are to control our stuttering as it exists now. From a practical standpoint, they are probably all that really matter. However, they do not necessarily explain how or why we began stuttering in the first place.

To discover the origins of stuttering, we must delve into deeper waters. Many possibilities must be explored: genetic factors, neurological factors, emotional factors, learned behavior, delays in speech development, parental attitudes toward speech, and so on. Although researchers have shed some light into these areas, the waters are still quite murky. There is no simple answer to why stuttering begins.

At the outset, we must distinguish between two types of stuttering with clearly different origins: *acquired stuttering* and *developmental stuttering*.

Acquired Stuttering

In a relatively few cases, the onset of stuttering can be traced to some kind of physical injury to the brain itself — perhaps caused by a blow to the head, a stroke, or other illness. This may occur at any age and is called **acquired stuttering**.

How brain damage may cause stuttering is not yet clear. Somehow, the brain's ability to select words or to produce speech might be physically disrupted, making speech more difficult. The person may adopt various struggle behaviors — including activation of the Valsalva mechanism — in an attempt to overcome the difficulty and force the words out. In this respect, the person with acquired stuttering may exhibit some of the same behaviors as other stutterers, even though the underlying cause of the disfluency is distinctly different.

Under extreme circumstances, stuttering might also begin at any age following a stressful or emotionally traumatic event, as sometimes happens to soldiers in battle. The adults who experience this may have had a previous history of stuttering when they were children.

Developmental Stuttering

The vast majority of stuttering does not involve any physical injury or severe emotional trauma. It just seems to arise of its own accord, for no particular reason. Because this kind of stuttering is often connected with the development of speech and language skills, some experts have called it **developmental stuttering**. This is the kind of stuttering to which this book is devoted.

Developmental stuttering usually begins in early childhood. At least 85 per cent of all cases begin between ages 2 and 8, with most starting somewhere between ages 3 and 5. The onset is usually gradual, progressing from simple disfluen-

Chapter 13 / The Origins of Stuttering

cies into more advanced forms of stuttering and avoidance behaviors.

Simple Disfluencies

A stutterer's first disfluencies are not usually what we would call stuttering. They are more like the simple disfluencies that many children exhibit during their speech development.

The child may hesitate, interject fillers like "umm" and "aah," and repeat whole words or phrases. He may say, for example, "Pass . . . pass . . . pass the potatoes."

Although the child is not totally fluent, he is not really stuttering either. He does not try to force out his words by using the Valsalva mechanism. His repetitions are easy, without the physical struggle and avoidance tactics usually seen in stuttering behavior.

Such disfluencies often occur when increased demands are placed on a child's speech and language abilities. Although he may have achieved fluency with simpler forms of speech, he is now confronted with longer words, more complicated sentence structure, complex rules of grammar and etiquette, and more difficult speaking situations. In addition, he must deal with subtle nuances of speech, such as inflection and intonation, that convey meanings beyond the words themselves.

The child, for whatever reason, may not be ready to meet these demands. It may take him a while to choose his words and to link them together in a grammatical sentence. While groping for words, he may fill in the gaps with interjections and repetitions to show that he hasn't stopped talking. (The same tactics are often used by normal adult speakers. Imagine, for example, a person trying to converse in a foreign language with which he is not totally familiar.)

In most children, these simple disfluencies are not viewed by the parents as being any cause for alarm. The disfluencies normally decrease as the child becomes more experienced in speaking. In other children, however, they may be more frequent and troublesome. There are several possible reasons for this.

Neurological factors. Some children may be delayed in their speech and language skills for various neurological reasons. For example, the speech centers of the brain may not have developed as quickly as in other children. The child may be slow in achieving the fine muscle coordination needed for speech. Consequently, his capacity for speech production may not be equal to the demands being made.

Studies show that stuttering children had been slower in their speech development, on the average, than non-stuttering children. But this is not true of all children who become stutterers. For example, the records of my childhood indicate that I had been quite advanced in my speaking skills before becoming disfluent.

Emotional factors. It is possible that the original disfluencies may have been triggered by anxiety or stress. Disfluency may suddenly appear, in some cases, after an emotionally disturbing event, going to a new school, a death or illness in the family, being left by parents with relatives or caretakers, marital discord between the parents, or other disruptions in the household. My own stuttering began during a time of stress at age 4, when my father was in the Army and my mother and I were forced to live with numerous relatives at my grandmother's house. Disfluency is also likely to increase when the child is excited.

Attitudes about speech. A child's difficulties can be aggravated if his parents or other adults put too much emphasis on the ability to speak well. In my own childhood situation, some of the grownups in the household had a habit of nitpicking at my speech. I was routinely scolded for bad grammar, using contractions (like "don't"), talking too loudly, or being rude. I lived in constant fear of "saying the wrong thing," and was warned that "a word once spoken can never be taken back." Speaking had all the perils of walking through a minefield.

The Progression of Stuttering

Some experts feel that the development of stuttering may be related to the child's inability to speak as well as his parents and other adults expect. If the disfluencies are felt to be excessive, the adults may show distress, annoyance, or concern. Studies show that parents have a tendency to speak more rapidly to a disfluent child and to interrupt him more often than other children.

The child may sense that his repetitions and interjections are slowing things down and making the adults impatient. Therefore, he may shorten and speed up his repetitions in an eagerness to get the words out more quickly. Starting with slower, less forceful repetitions of longer units (whole words), he may progress to more rapid repetitions of shorter units (part-words and beginning sounds) with more force. (This is described by Starkweather, 1987.)

For example, instead of repeating the whole word "pass," the child may repeat only the first consonant and vowel, so it comes out, "Pa . . . pa . . . pa . . . pass the potatoes."

As the child further shortens the repeated unit and speeds up the repetition, he will begin to say, "Puh-puh-puh-pass." Notice how the proper vowel (*a*) has been replaced in the repeated segment by *uh*. This is known as the **schwa**. It is a neutral sound that comes out when we are not trying to pronounce any vowel in particular. The next step would be to drop the *schwa* and simply repeat the consonant very rapidly, as in "P-p-p-p-pass."

This progression can go still further by focusing on even smaller parts of the consonant itself. For example, the *p* sound is formed by (1) closing the lips to cause a slight build-up of air pressure; and then (2) opening the lips to release a puff of air. The child may repeat only the *closure* part of the consonant, without the release, resulting in a prolonged blockage of air.

Air Pressure and Force

This scenario shows how slow, easy repetitions of whole words can progress into rapid repetitions of smaller units and finally into a complete stuttering block. While the child's original motive may have been to produce the words more quickly, what actually results is a tendency *to build up air pressure and to increase the amount of force.*

In the word "pass," for example, the greatest air pressure is concentrated on the initial plosive, *p*. When the plosive is released, the air pressure decreases. However, if you skip the rest of the word and repeat the *p* sound rapidly, the air pressure will continue to build up. The more rapid the repetition and the smaller the segment being repeated, the more air pressure is sustained. During a prolonged closure, the air pressure would be greatest of all.

The same is true when the child repeats an initial vowel sound (as in *apple*). As previously discussed, we typically close the vocal cords and false vocal cords to block air flow before an initial vowel. We let the air pressure build up slightly and then release it, in order to accentuate the beginning of the vowel sound. Here the air pressure is built up by closure of the larynx instead of the mouth.

During this progression, the child may learn to associate the feeling of air pressure with his efforts to get the words out. This is where the body's Valsalva mechanism comes into play. It is specifically designed to build up air pressure in the lungs by tightening the chest and abdominal muscles, while forcefully closing the mouth or larynx to keep air from escaping. The greater the air pressure, the more forcefully the mouth or larynx closes.

This process is the Valsalva maneuver, with which we are now familiar. Since it is the same maneuver that the child previously relied upon to help him in defecation and other types of physical effort, it is highly plausible that he would use it in his attempt to force out words. As a result, the Valsalva mechanism would increase the force with which he closes his mouth or larynx, as well as the amount of air pressure. It would give him the illusion that he is "trying hard" to produce the words and to please his impatient parents and other adults.

Once the Valsalva mechanism gets involved, the child's disfluency takes on a whole new character. As we have seen, the neurological tuning of the Valsalva mechanism may interfere with the ability to phonate and may increase the likelihood of excessively forceful closures of the mouth and larynx. Therefore, the harder he tries to force the words out, the more his speech is blocked.

Unlike the earlier disfluencies, the child's stuttering is now more likely to become focused on specific words or speaking situations. He will learn to anticipate difficulty and to activate the Valsalva mechanism in order to force the words out, resulting in the very difficulty he feared. He may then adopt various secondary behaviors in an attempt to avoid, postpone, break through, or hide the stuttering blocks.

Before long, the child may find himself caught in the Valsalva-Stuttering Cycle previously described. This will tend to perpetuate the stuttering indefinitely, even if the original cause for the disfluency disappears.

The Crucial Question of Recovery

Nevertheless, it is a significant fact that at least half of all children who begin stuttering will become reasonably fluent by the time they reach age 16, even without therapy. This is called **spontaneous recovery**. Some experts have suggested that the crucial difference between stutterers and fluents may not lie so much in the original disfluencies or stuttering, but in the capacity *to recover* from stuttering.

Studies show that 75 per cent of those stuttering at age 4 and 50 per cent of those stuttering at age 6 will be better by age 16. However, if the child is still stuttering at age 10, his likelihood of spontaneous recovery drops to only 25 per cent.

There seems to be a crucial period between ages 5 and 7 during which speech patterns become fixed. If a child continues to stutter during this period, the stuttering behavior will become firmly established and difficult to change. Therefore, stuttering should be treated as soon as possible, before it passes this critical phase.

The ability to recover from stuttering may also vary according to sex. Some studies indicate that the simple disfluencies of early childhood are almost as common among girls as among boys. However, the girls are more likely than boys to recover. (It is also interesting to note that girls who are right handed are more likely to recover than girls who are left handed.) When we come to chronic stutterers, males greatly outnumber females by estimated ratios of at least 3 to 1 (and perhaps as high as 5 to 1).

Sex Differences and the Valsalva Mechanism

What can account for this striking disparity between males and females in the prevalence of stuttering? Is there some physical, neurological, or behavioral difference that might be responsible?

Various explanations have been offered for this differential. Some experts have proposed a sex-linked hereditary factor. Others have attributed it to the general tendency of boys to be slower in their speech development than girls, and therefore more likely to have difficulty in expressing themselves verbally. Or it may be due to a combination of factors.

The Valsalva Hypothesis opens up yet another avenue of investigation, based on the possibility of *sexual differences in the Valsalva mechanism.*

The Valsalva mechanism is common to both sexes. It is particularly important to women during natural childbirth, because the Valsalva maneuver helps to push the baby out of the uterus. However, the Valsalva mechanism seems to have developed to a greater extent in men, possibly because of its use in the kinds of strenuous physical activities that men have traditionally performed.

The larynx — a key part of the Valsalva mechanism — is significantly larger in men than in women, as evidenced by the familiar "Adam's Apple" that bulges out the front of a man's throat. This characteristic allows the larynx to perform effort closure more forcefully during a Valsalva maneuver, so as to retain greater air pressure in the lungs.

In view of these physical distinctions in the Valsalva mechanisms of men and women, it would not be surprising to find neurological differences as well. Such differences might exist in children, even before the larynx increases in size during puberty. To the extent that boys are more physically active than girls, they may be more accustomed to performing Valsalva maneuvers while exerting effort. Consequently, boys might have a greater tendency to use the Valsalva mechanism when trying to overcome difficulties in speech.

Genetic Factors

There is evidence that stuttering may be linked to genetic factors in approximately half the persons who stutter. As we shall see in Chapter 15, a child is more likely to stutter if he or she has a close relative who does. Also, the correlation of stuttering is much greater between identical twins than between fraternal twins.

However, genetic factors are obviously not the whole story. While they may be involved in determining the *likelihood* of some children stuttering, genetic factors do not seem to have any correlation to how often or how *severely* a child will stutter. Furthermore, the most significant genetic factors seem to be less related to the original disfluencies than to the question of whether the child will be among the 75 per cent who *recover* from stuttering spontaneously or among the 25 per cent who *persist* in stuttering.

Assuming that there is a genetic predisposition to stutter, it is not conclusive that the genes will in fact cause stuttering to occur. It is also unclear as to what exactly the genetic tendency would be. Is it a tendency to repeat? To hesitate? To force? And how might these factors be related to the speech functions of the brain and the ability of a person to recover from stuttering?

These and other questions will be explored in subsequent chapters.

General References

AMBROSE, N. G., COX, N. J., & YAIRI, E. The genetic basis of persistence and recovery in stuttering. *Journal of Speech, Language and Hearing Research,* 1997, 40, 567-80.

ANDREWS, G., CRAIG, A., FEYER, A., HODDINOTT, S., HOWIE, P., & NEILSON, M. Stuttering: a review of research findings and theories circa 1982. *Journal of Speech and Hearing Disorders,* 1983, 48, 226-246.

BLOODSTEIN, O. *A Handbook on Stuttering.* 5th ed. San Diego: Singular Publishing Group, 1995, pp. 105-272, 359-392.

FINK, B. R. The curse of Adam: Effort closure of the larynx. *Anesthesiology,* 1973, 39, 325-327.

JOHNSON, W., ET AL. *The Onset of Stuttering.* Minneapolis: University of Michigan Press, 1959.

JOHNSON, W., ET AL. A study of the onset and development of stuttering. *Stuttering Then and Now* (edited by Shames, G.H., & Rubin, H.). Columbus, OH: Charles E. Merrill Publishing Co., 1986, 125-129.

KEHOE, T. D. *Stuttering: Science, Therapy & Practice.* Boulder, CO: Casa Futura Technologies, 1999, 38-41.

PETERS, T. J., & GUITAR, B. *Stuttering: An Integrated Approach to Its Nature and Treatment.* Baltimore: Williams & Wilkins, 1991, pp. 43-107.

SMITH, A. Factors in the etiology of stuttering. *Research Needs in Stuttering: Roadblocks and Future Directions. ASHA Reports,* 1990, 18, 39-47.

STARKWEATHER, C. W. *Fluency and Stuttering.* Englewood Cliffs, N.J.: Prentice-Hall, 1987, pp. 37-47, 137-167.

VAN RIPER, C. *The Nature of Stuttering.* 2nd ed. Englewood Cliffs, N.J.: Prentice-Hall, 1982, pp. 58-110.

YAIRI, E., AMBROSE, N. G., & COX, N. J. Genetics of stuttering: a critical review. *Journal of Speech and Hearing Research,* 1996, 39, 771-84.

CHAPTER 14.

Speech Functions of the Brain

OUR SEARCH FOR THE ORIGIN of stuttering ultimately leads to that infinitely complex and mysterious organ, the brain. Here are located the processing areas that translate words into detailed motor programs for speech, as well as the command centers that activate the appropriate muscles of the larynx, mouth, and respiratory system. This is also where the plans go awry — where phonation is supplanted by Valsalva tuning and excessive force, and fluency is replaced by stuttering.

How and why might this happen? Is there something peculiar about a stutterer's brain that creates a tendency to stutter? Are there physical or neurological factors that make it difficult for the stutterer to overcome the disfluencies of early childhood, as discussed in the previous chapter?

To help us explore these questions more fully, we will quickly review the brain's structure and its areas devoted to speech and language.

Brain Matter

Our brain is an intricate network of more than 100 billion nerve cells, called **neurons**. They come in many varieties, designed for particular purposes.

Basically, each neuron has a cell body covered with hundreds or even thousands of branching fibers called **dendrites**. These are lined with little bulbs, called **spines**, which receive signals from other neurons. The neuron also has a long fiber called an **axon**, through which it sends impulses *to* other neurons.

The axon is often covered with a fatty sheath called **myelin**, which helps to speed up the transmission of nerve impulses. Because the myelin is white in appearance, those portions of the brain that carry many axons are called **white matter**. The areas containing a heavy concentration of nerve bodies and dendrites are called **gray matter**.

Each axon has many branches at its far end, which connect to the spines on the dendrites or cell bodies of other neurons. The connection is called a **synapse**. The brain may have as many as *one quadrillion* synaptic connections in all.

Inside the neuron, signals travel as electrical impulses. But when they get to a synapse, the signals have to cross a **synaptic cleft**, which is about a millionth of an inch wide. Here the signal is passed along by means of special chemicals, called **neurotransmitters**.

These chemicals are released by a specialized knob called a **synaptic terminal**, located at the end of the axon branch. The chemicals travel across the synaptic cleft and enter the spines on the receiving neuron. Here they create an electrical

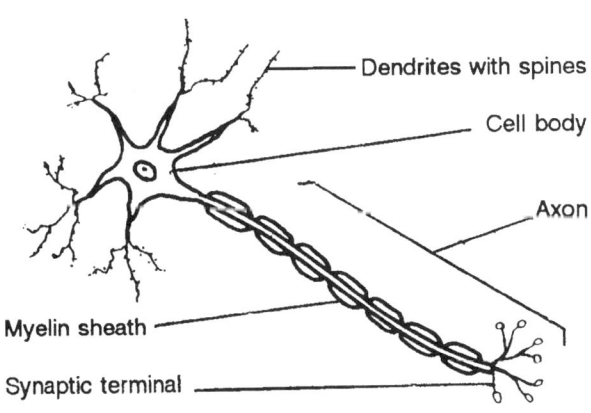

SIMPLIFIED DIAGRAM OF A NEURON

charge, which travels to the cell body.

When the total signals received by a neuron add up to a certain **threshold level**, the cell will fire an electrical impulse, which travels down its axon to the synapses where it connects to other neurons. In this way, nerve impulses are relayed from neuron to neuron, throughout the brain and to the muscles of the body. The routes that the impulses follow are called **nerve pathways**.

Anatomy of the Brain

The neurons are organized into a number of larger structures within the brain, each with specialized functions of its own. By far the largest of these structures is the **cerebrum**, which fills the top of the head. About the size of a small melon, its surface is wrinkled like a walnut's. It is split down the middle into two halves, called **hemispheres** — the left and the right — separated by a deep valley called the **longitudinal fissure**.

The surface of the cerebrum is folded into numerous ridges (**gyri**) and grooves (**fissures** or **sulci**). This design allows a large amount of surface area to be squeezed inside the skull. The surface is covered by a thin layer of gray matter called the **cerebral cortex**. The cortex contains nerve centers dealing with sight and hearing, voluntary movement, and higher mental functions, including language and speech.

Beneath the cerebral cortex are vast areas of white matter, containing bundles of axons that connect the cortex with other parts of the brain and nervous system. These include a bridge of nerve fibers, called the **corpus callosum**, which connects the two hemispheres.

Circling the innermost part of the cerebrum is a group of structures called the **limbic system**. This area is the seat of our emotions and other basic, animal drives. Beneath this are several masses of gray matter called the **basal ganglia**. They serve as relay stations for motor impulses passing between the cortex and other areas. Wedged under the back of the cerebrum is a cauliflower-shaped structure called the **cerebellum**, or "little brain," which helps to coordinate the movements of our body.

The **brainstem** forms the base of the brain. It controls many bodily functions, such as respiration. It also provides a pathway from the brain to the

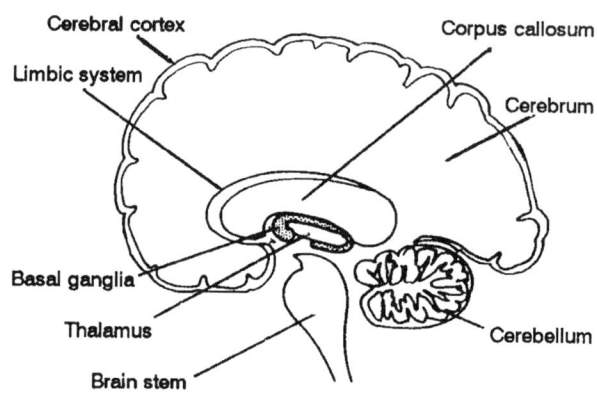

MID-SECTION OF THE BRAIN

body, since it is the source of the **cranial nerves** (which operate the mouth and larynx) and it leads to the **spinal cord** (which controls the respiratory muscles and the rest of the body).

Speech Centers of the Brain

The principal centers for speech and language are almost always located on one side of the brain, which is referred to as the **dominant hemisphere**. This is on the *left side* in about 95 per cent of all people (including 99 per cent of right-handers and many left-handers as well). Therefore, we shall refer to the left hemisphere as being dominant for the purpose of our discussion.

Most of the language centers are found in a region along the side of the dominant hemisphere known as the **perisylvian zone**. This zone contains a number of **association areas**, where we think about what we want to say and make the initial decision to speak.

Another center of particular importance is **Wernicke's area**, which is located slightly above and behind the left ear. It helps us to understand language and to arrange our thoughts into intelligible words and sentences.

Once the words have been properly put together in Wernicke's area, the signals travel forward in the brain, along a bundle of nerve fibers called the **arcuate fasciculus**, to a speech center known as **Broca's area**. This is located slightly above and to the front of the ear. Here the brain matches up the words with a detailed "motor program" for moving the appropriate muscles of our

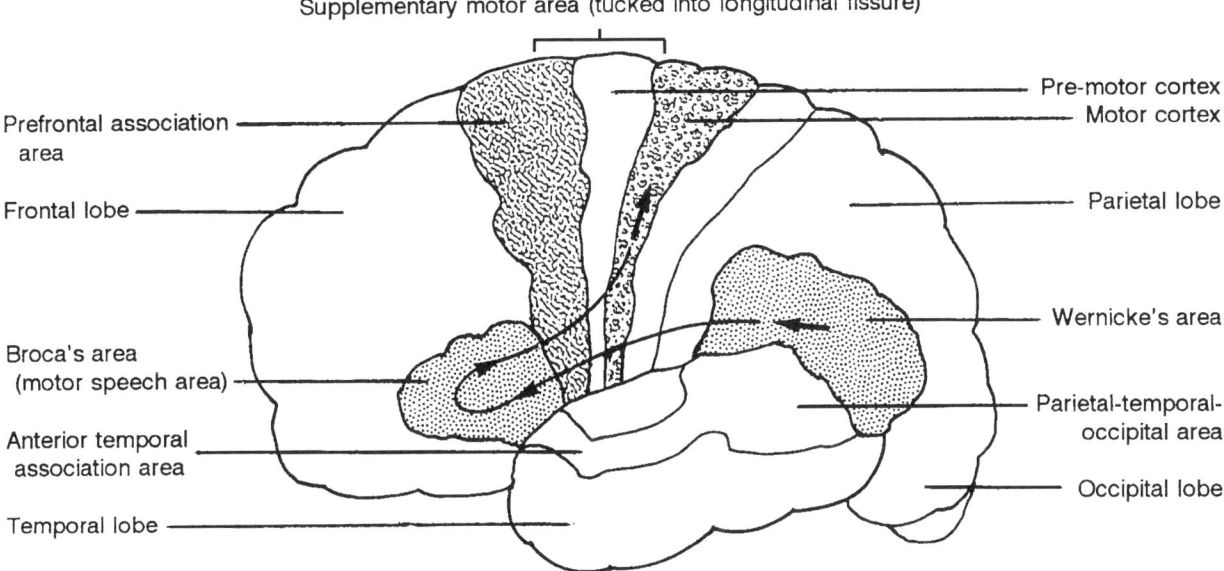

Arrowed line represents the route traveled by speech signals, including the arcuate fasciculus.

SPEECH AREAS OF THE BRAIN

speech mechanism in just the right sequence.

The signals are then sent to the **motor cortex**, which forms a strip arching over the top of the head. The motor cortex sends signals to the larynx, lips, tongue, and respiratory muscles to prepare for and execute the movements necessary for speech. Assisting in the preparations for speech is a strip known as the **premotor area**, just in front of the motor cortex, and the **supplementary motor area**, tucked inside the longitudinal fissure at the top of the head.

There is also a small, third speech area, found at the top of the dominant hemisphere, slightly to the front of the motor cortex, called the **supplemental speech area**. During normal speech, all of these areas seem to interact with and assist one another in the production of speech.

The **non-dominant hemisphere** (usually the *right side*) may make its own contributions to speech. The right hemisphere contains the area for music. It may supply the musical aspects of our speech — such as intonation, inflection, rhythm, and emotional expression. The right hemisphere may also have a limited amount of language ability. This is particularly true with regard to simple, emotionally charged words — such as the swear words and other exclamations we might utter when emotionally aroused.

It is interesting to note that persons with severe aphasia, who are unable to speak because of damage to the left hemisphere, may still be able to sing or to shout expletives - indicating that these functions are preserved in the right brain.

The Interaction of Many Parts

The production of speech does not simply move through the brain in a linear fashion, like automobiles on an assembly line. It is an organic process in which many parts interact, with each part influencing every other part. Speech also involves many structures in the brain besides the cerebral cortex.

The limbic system provides the underlying drives that motivate our speech. The basal ganglia act as relay stations between the association areas and other parts of the brain. In addition, the basal ganglia may facilitate the movements of speech by inhibiting other types of motor activity that might interfere.

The **thalamus**, located in the brainstem, may coordinate the activities of Broca's and Wernicke's areas. Some researchers believe that the thalamus also participates somehow in timing, initiating movement, modulating speech, and controlling respiration. The cerebellum helps to coordinate the rapid and precise movements of articulation, as well as the smooth transition from one position to the next.

The Effect of Experience

The brain, unlike a computer, is a living organ. Although the number of brain cells does not increase after early childhood, our experiences and behavior can profoundly affect the number of synaptic connections within the brain — and, consequently, its ability to function. As we engage in new activities, the neurons' dendrites, spines, and synaptic terminals grow and make new contacts. This is particularly important during the early years of life, when the child is learning new skills and the brain is physically growing in size. However, the process continues to some extent throughout our lives.

When we first learn a new skill, the neurons grope around, trying to form nerve pathways to those parts of the brain and the body that must participate in the necessary actions. Like explorers cutting a path through the wilderness, the neurons may go through a lot of trial and error as they look for the right connections. As we continue to practice, the nerve pathways become stronger and more efficient. With repeated use, the path becomes a road and then a highway.

The more we engage in a particular activity, the more neurons and nerve pathways will become devoted to that type of behavior. Some skills, like riding a bicycle or throwing a ball, may become so habitual that we never forget them. Their nerve pathways are preserved in the network of neurons, axons, and dendrites in some part of the brain. Conversely, an activity that we neglect will have fewer neurons, fewer synaptic contacts, and weaker nerve pathways at its disposal.

Nerve Pathways and Stuttering

The same principle applies to speech. The more we talk, the stronger become the pathways that link the speech centers of the brain and the organs of speech. This fact may have an enormous impact on the speech development of a person who stutters.

If a child's early disfluencies inhibit him from talking, his speech experience will be somewhat limited. Consequently, the speech areas of his brain may not develop as fully as in a child who speaks more often. This deficiency would be further complicated if he learns to build up air pressure, by using the Valsalva mechanism, in an effort to force out his words.

By repeatedly performing a Valsalva maneuver while struggling to talk, he will establish strong nerve pathways from the brain's speech centers to the Valsalva mechanism. If this behavior continues during the formative years of brain development (especially during ages 5 to 7), these pathways may become permanently ingrained, at the expense of the pathways for phonation and fluent speech. As a result, the speech functions of his brain may remain chronically weak and subject to interference in times of stress. He will have a neurological tendency to tune his Valsalva mechanism, causing difficulty in phonation, excessively forceful closures, and other forms of stuttering behavior.

In the next chapter, we shall discuss the question of whether the brain of a person who stutters is somehow different from that of a fluent person. We shall explore the extent to which stuttering may be influenced by heredity or various neurological conditions.

General References

BEATON, A. *Left Side, Right Side: A Review of Laterality Research.* New Haven: Yale University Press, 1985.
DIMOND, S. J. *Neuropsychology.* London: Butterworths, 1980.
HOOPER, J. & DICK, T. *The Three-Pound Universe.* New York: MacMillan Publishing Co., 1986.
LOVE, R. J. & WEBB, W. G. *Neurology for the Speech-Language Pathologist.* Stoneham, MA: Butterworth, 1986.
NOBACK, C. R., STROMINGER, N.L., & DEMAREST, R. J. *The Human Nervous System: Introduction and Review.* 4th ed. New York: McGraw-Hill Book Co., 1991.
SCIENTIFIC AMERICAN. *The Brain.* New York: W. H. Freeman & Co., 1979.
THOMPSON, R. F. *The Brain: An Introduction to Neuroscience.* New York: W. H. Freeman & Co., 1985.

CHAPTER 15.

Heredity and the Stutterer's Brain

STUTTERING CANNOT be fully explained by learned behavior or psychological and environmental influences. We must look elsewhere to determine why some people are more susceptible to stuttering than others. Many speech scientists believe that the tendency to stutter is inherited through abnormalities in the structure or chemistry of the brain.

This possibility has profound implications for persons who stutter. Many of us welcome the idea that stuttering has an inherited, organic basis, rather than purely psychological causes, because it frees us from the stigma of "mental illness" and personal guilt. We can stop blaming ourselves for our failed attempts at fluency. The fault lies not in ourselves, so to speak, but in our genes.

On the other hand, it is depressing — and inaccurate — to think of ourselves as helpless victims of a brain defect. Just because stuttering is not our "fault" does not mean that it is totally beyond our control. If we can understand exactly *what* the defect is and *how* it promotes stuttering, perhaps we can develop an effective strategy to improve fluency in spite of it.

In this chapter, we shall address important questions about the hereditary factor in stuttering and the types of neurological defects that might be involved.

Is the Risk of Stuttering Inherited?

The existence of an inherited predisposition toward chronic stuttering is supported by genetic studies, which show an increased risk among people with close relatives who stutter. On the other hand, approximately one-half of all chronic stutterers have *no* stuttering relatives — indicating that genetics might *not* be a factor for those individuals.

The risk is by far the greatest if the stuttering relative is your *identical twin* — a person whose genetic makeup is exactly the same as yours. If one identical twin stutters, the chances are at least 58 per cent that the other twin will also stutter. (Some studies report correlations of up to 90 per cent.) In contrast, the correlation of stuttering between *fraternal* twins (those who are not genetically identical) is only about 13 per cent.

While these findings may seem impressive, they must be viewed with caution. To some extent, the prevalence of stuttering within certain families may reflect a similarity of environmental factors and attitudes about speech. This is especially true in the case of identical twins — who are often treated alike and who tend to identify closely with one another. It should not be surprising that both might fall into the same habits of speech.

For a truer measure of the genetic factor, we would need to compare stuttering in sets of identical twins who were *separated at birth* and grew up in different families. In the only such study of which I am aware, a researcher found *no* correlation of stuttering based on five sets of identical twins who were separated at birth. In each case, only *one* of the twins stuttered; the other did not. (Farber, 1981.)

A recent study indicates that genetic factors may play a greater role in chronic stutterers who are *female* than those who are male. When you consider only those chronic stutterers *who have relatives who stutter*, the male-to-female ratio is only 1.57-to-one (or approximately 60% to 40%), as compared to approximately four-to-one (or 80% to 20%) in the general stuttering population. In contrast, those chronic stutterers who *don't* have stuttering relatives are overwhelmingly *male*. (Drayna, et al., 1999.) If the above figures hold true, they indicate that heredity is much more likely to be a factor in female chronic stutterers than in males.

Even when genetic factors are present, it is clear that they do not necessarily condemn us to stutter. Nor do they seem to control how *frequently* or *severely* we will stutter. They only increase the *likelihood* that we will do so.

Whether this likelihood actually turns into stuttering may depend on other factors, discussed in previous chapters. We may *learn* certain habits (such as trying to "force out" words when we anticipate difficulty in speaking) which themselves interfere with speech and become self-perpetuating through a vicious circle. If these behaviors continue through the formative years of childhood, they may leave a lasting imprint on the nerve pathways of the brain.

What Traits Are Crucial to Stuttering?

Merely saying that we may inherit a "tendency to stutter" leaves many questions unanswered. What exactly *is* the crucial trait, and how does it promote stuttering?

Some people might assume that stutterers simply inherit the more obvious *symptoms* of stuttering — for example, the tendency to repeat, to prolong sounds, or to block. But this type of behavior, *in and of itself*, is probably not the trait that distinguishes stutterers from other people.

Stuttering-like disfluencies are not unique to stutterers, and they are not necessarily abnormal. Almost anyone may occasionally hesitate, repeat or prolong sounds, or even block on a word. This behavior is quite common when people are afraid, confused, excited, or struggling to converse in an unfamiliar language. It is often seen in children, during certain stages of speech development. These simple forms of stuttering may simply be a natural reaction to circumstances that interfere with the flow of speech.

A more extreme example of this behavior is seen in **acquired stutterers** — previously normal speakers who suddenly began to stutter after physical damage to the brain, caused by injury or disease. In view of the fact that acquired stutterers generally have no family history of stuttering, they provide dramatic evidence that stuttering-like behavior can exist in *anyone* — without the need for a genetic factor.

The same is probably true of **developmental stutterers**, who began stuttering as children and then went on to become chronic stutterers as they got older. If they have a genetic defect, it is probably not the stuttering itself, but something less obvious that *promotes* stuttering.

Some experts propose that the trait may involve delays in language development or defects in coordination. Others believe that the fundamental difference between chronic stutterers and nonstutterers is the *inability to overcome the early forms of stuttering that most children outgrow*. It has been suggested that chronic stutterers may have inherited characteristics that allow stuttering to persist during their formative years and to become deeply rooted in the nerve pathways of speech.

As previously noted, the ability to spontaneously recover from stuttering is also related to a child's sex. Although the ratio between boy and girl stutterers is about equal when they are very young, a much higher percentage of the girls recover than boys. Consequently, the boys who persist in stuttering eventually outnumber the girls by a ratio of at least four to one. Those girls who *don't* recover are more likely to have relatives who stutter.

Does the Stutterer's Brain Have a Physical Defect?

Whatever the inherited characteristic might be, it has not shown up as an identifiable defect in the *physical structure* of the brain. Diagnostic tests such as X-rays, CAT scans, and MRI scans have not revealed any specific physical abnormality that causes developmental stuttering. MRI studies have shown, however, that stutterers may have a greater number of atypical anatomical features in the speech areas of the brain than fluent speakers have. Such anomolies might increase the *risk* of stuttering. (Foundas.)

While specific physical brain defects might show up in isolated cases, they are not common to developmental stutterers in general. They might not even be inherited. Usually, physical defects are only visible in the brains of *acquired* stutterers and represent *non*-inherited damage caused by injury or disease.

By studying the location of brain damage in

Chapter 15 / Heredity and the Stutterer's Brain

acquired stutterers, some researchers have hoped to pinpoint places in the brain that might be related to developmental stuttering as well. However, this hasn't been easy. The visible areas of damage, called **lesions**, have not been confined to a particular area, but have been found in many different locations. In other cases, the stuttering has followed a **diffuse brain injury**, in which the force of the impact was spread throughout the *entire* brain.

Consequently, there is no single spot in the brain that must be injured in order to cause stuttering. More likely, the acquired stutterers' injuries simply make speech *more difficult* by damaging any of a number of different parts of the brain that interact during speech. The stuttering-like behavior may then appear as a natural response to the difficulty.

If increased difficulty in speaking can trigger stuttering-like responses in acquired stutterers, this might also be true in developmental stutterers. However, they probably do not have the kind of brain damage found in acquired stutterers. There are significant differences between the symptoms of developmental and acquired stuttering, which indicate that the underlying difficulties are not the same.

The disfluencies of acquired stuttering reflect a *constant neurological impairment*, not subject to the emotional factors and other variables that affect developmental stuttering. Acquired stutterers usually don't experience anxiety or anticipation about certain words or speaking situations. Instead of blocking mainly at the beginnings of words and sentences, like developmental stutterers, they tend to stutter uniformly throughout their speech.

No matter how many times an acquired stutterer reads the same passage over and over, his fluency is not likely to improve, whereas developmental stutterers usually become more fluent after repeated practice (a phenomenon known as the **adaptation effect**). Furthermore, an acquired stutterer's brain damage may cause other neurological problems (such as difficulty in putting words together or coordinating movement) to an extent not usually found in developmental stutterers.

Therefore, developmental stuttering must involve factors that are more complex and variable than mere physical damage to the brain.

Do Stutterers' Brains Function Differently?

Another way to search for the distinguishing characteristic is to look for abnormalities in the way a stutterer's brain *functions*. Brain defects are sometimes indicated by irregularities in the brain's electrical impulses (or "brain waves"), by the amount of blood flow to various parts of the brain, and by its response to various stimuli. Although the studies are often conflicting, some scientists have found evidence that stutterers' brains operate differently than those of normal speakers.

Patterns of brain activity. During the past several years, researchers have been using sophisticated diagnostic equipment to produce computerized pictures showing subtle differences in the patterns of activity in stutterers' brains.

One widely used method is **positron emission tomography** ("PET"). After radioactive tracers are injected into a person's bloodstream, a PET camera is used to detect the emission of positrons (positive electrons) from various parts of the brain. The emission of positrons indicates which parts of the brain are most active, based on such things as relative blood flow or consumption of sugar.

PET scans are first taken of the brain while the person is at rest or performing some baseline mental activity. Then PET scans are taken during or immediately after the performance of specific verbal or auditory tasks. The computer then subtracts out the baseline results to show the relative degree to which various parts of the brain are more or less active as compared to baseline.

Although each person's PET scan is unique, the computer combines the scans of numerous individuals to come up with an average group pattern. The computer then compares the group pattern of stutterers with that of non-stutterers to show how their brain activity differs during the performance of various tasks. To highlight the differences, the PET scan pictures usually show the relative degrees of activity in contrasting colors.

There have been a number of PET studies, using different methods, subjects, and equipment, and the results have not been totally consistent. Compared to non-stutterers, most studies showed that stutterers, as a group, had *slightly less activity* around the speech areas on the left side of the brain and more activity on the *right* side of the brain. While stuttering, the stutterers also had decreased activity in the auditory regions and diffuse overactivity in various motor areas. Many of these abnormalities were reduced or eliminated when stutterers spoke fluently under fluency-enhancing conditions (such as choral reading).

Some researchers have focused on an area in the basal ganglia called the **left striatum** or **caudate**, which appears to have reduced activity in stutterers during both stuttered and fluent speech. (Wu, Maguire, et al., 1995.) In comparison to non-stutterers, stutterers were also found to have a significantly higher uptake of **dopamine** (a neurotransmitter) in certain parts of the brain that modulate verbalization. (Wu, Maguire, et al., 1997.) Those researchers have hypothesized that dopamine might be responsible for inhibiting activity in those areas of the brain.

The meaning of these findings is uncertain. Because PET scans are not permitted on small children, it is unclear whether differences in brain function were the original *cause* of stuttering, or whether they are instead the *effect* of many years of stuttering behavior. It is possible that stutterers' nerve pathways for normal speech are weak because of relative disuse, while the nerve pathways for force and struggle have been strengthened by constant use. If such is the case, it should be no surprise that stutterers have developed inappropriate patterns of brain activity.

Hemispheric dominance. In the vast majority of people, the processing of speech is **lateralized** — that is, concentrated in one hemisphere of the brain or the other. The hemisphere containing the speech center is referred to as being **dominant**. Using a variety of neurological tests, researchers have found that nearly all right-handers and about two-thirds of the left-handers have their speech centers on the *left side* of the brain. In other people (primarily left-handers), speech processing may be either on the right side or on *both* sides — a condition known as **bilateral speech**.

According to some studies, *a majority of stutterers show evidence of bilateral speech*. In fact, the amount of speech activity in the right hemisphere seems to increase in proportion to the severity of stuttering. It is not known whether a stutterer's bilateral speech is inherited or learned.

Some studies have shown that when a stutterer becomes more fluent through therapy, the speech activity tends to shift back to the left hemisphere.

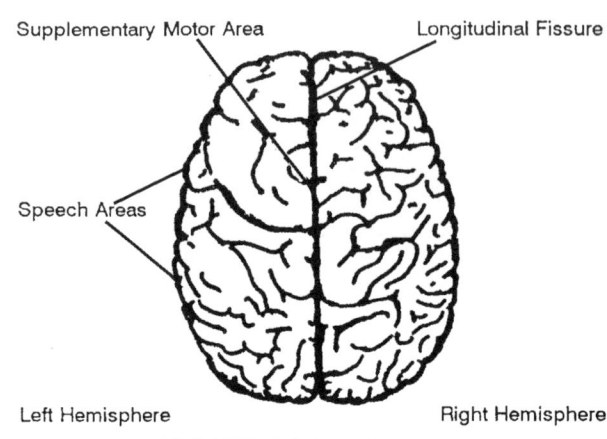

TOP VIEW OF THE BRAIN

However, even after intensive fluency shaping therapy, the lateralization of brain function may not be totally normalized. (De Nil, 1998.)

These facts have raised speculation that stuttering may somehow result from a lack of hemispheric dominance. The left hemisphere is usually superior in performing tasks that involve a rapid sequence of movements, such as speech. Therefore, some experts say that the left hemisphere must be dominant in order to give proper timing and coordination to the muscles of speech.

Even if hemispheric dominance plays some role, the mere presence of bilateral speech cannot be the determining factor in all cases of stuttering. Many stutterers *don't* have bilateral speech, and the great majority of people with bilateral speech don't stutter. Furthermore, we still must explain the variability of stuttering within each individual. Could it be that the brain's right hemisphere interacts with some *other* factor (such as the Valsalva mechanism) to cause these symptoms?

Do Stutterers Have Neurological Deficiencies?

Still another approach to finding the inherited defect is to look for deficiencies in the way stutterers perform on various neurological tests. Over the years, many researchers have reported that stutterers, as a group, tend to show poorer-than-average performance on a number of levels. Here are some of the aspects in which differences have been found.

Intelligence and language skills. Some researchers tell us that stutterers, on the average, perform significantly worse than the general population on tests of intelligence and language skills. In addition, the risk of stuttering is three times greater than average in the mentally retarded. (On the other hand, stutterers who are in therapy seem to be *more* intelligent than average.)

Some of these findings may come as a shock to people active in the stuttering community, who have nurtured the idea that stutterers tend to be pretty bright. Indeed, some of history's greatest thinkers and writers have stuttered — people like Sir Isaac Newton, Charles Darwin, Sir Winston Churchill, Charles Lamb, Lewis Carroll, and W. Somerset Maugham, to name a few.

Clearly, stuttering is not caused by, nor is it a sign of low intelligence. However, it is possible that people of lower intelligence are more prone to delays in language development, which may add to the *difficulty* of speech and thereby promote stuttering. In other words, these deficits may increase the *risk* of stuttering, but they certainly are not necessary or determining factors.

Reaction speed. Studies show that stutterers are not as quick in their reaction time as nonstutterers. For example, when asked to press a button in response to a signal, stutterers take a few milliseconds longer, on the average, than normal speakers. When a vocal response is required (such as making a vowel sound while exhaling), the delay is even greater.

Some speech pathologists interpret these results as indicating a defect in the way a stutterer's brain processes motor commands. These deficiencies are more pronounced in children than adults. Therefore, they may have more to do with the *original disfluencies* of childhood than with the chronic stuttering of later years.

An interesting finding is that adult stutterers, unlike normal speakers, can make a voiced sound more quickly while *inhaling* than while exhaling. We must look to the involvement of some *other* factor — such as the Valsalva mechanism — to explain this phenomenon.

Coordination and timing of movement. Researchers have tested stutterers' skills in activating and coordinating fine movements, such as rapid finger maneuvers and putting pegs in holes. Again, stutterers don't do quite as well as normal speakers. These results may suggest a neurological deficiency that affects more than just speech. Some researchers have suggested the possibility of weakness in the brain's **supplementary motor area**.

The coordination of a stutterer's speech is, of course, severely disrupted during stuttering. But some speech pathologists report that stutterers continue to show subtle defects in coordination, even when they seem fluent. For example, sensitive instruments may indicate that a stutterer's phonation is slightly delayed or poorly coordinated with airflow and articulation. Other researchers have found *no* significant abnormalities when stutterers speak fluently.

While a slight deficiency in coordination may tend to make speech *more difficult*, this would not necessarily cause stuttering. Regardless of the neurological deficits that might exist, they obviously can't be so bad if a stutterer is capable of speech that at least *sounds* fluent. The problem is not that stutterers *lack* the neurological capacity to coordinate speech, but rather that some force *interferes* with their ability to do so. Any signs of discoordination in a stutterer's fluent speech might simply indicate a residual amount of interference.

The question remains as to *what* the interfering force is, and *why* it interferes more at some times than at others.

Control over laryngeal reflexes. Using fiberoptic tubes and electrodes, researchers have observed abnormal behavior in the larynx during stuttering. In addition to forcefully closing the airway, the laryngeal muscles may contract in various other ways that are inappropriate to phonation. These movements are involuntary and cannot be duplicated when the stutterer is asked to stutter on purpose.

Some experts think this behavior might be caused by automatic reflexes, stimulated by changes in air pressure during speech. They have suggested that a stutterer's brain may be *deficient in its ability to inhibit reflexes* of the larynx that may interfere with phonation. (This might suggest a defect in the **basal ganglia**, which are normally responsible for suppressing inappropriate reflexes.)

But changes in air pressure *always* occur during speech. Why, then, would the interfering reflexes tend to occur only *some* of the time? Again, the missing piece to this puzzle may be the Valsalva mechanism.

Although not mentioned by the experts, the

reflexes of the Valsalva mechanism could explain some of this behavior. During **effort closure**, the laryngeal muscles tighten in response to air pressure, thereby blocking the airway and interfering with phonation. The activation of the Valsalva mechanism would be *variable*, depending on how much we anticipate that speaking will be difficult. Furthermore, Valsalva tuning may also have the neurological effect of increasing other reflex activity (as we shall discuss in the next chapter).

Neuropsychological subgroups. Adding further complexity to the problem is the possibility that neurological weaknesses are not the same in all stutterers. Researchers in Edmonton, Alberta, put stutterers through a battery of neuropsychological tests, which revealed differences not only in the severity of their deficits, but also in the areas of the brain that seemed to be involved.

The tests indicated deficiencies in such areas as the brainstem, left midbrain, thalamus, frontal lobes, pre-motor cortex, motor cortex, supplementary motor area, Broca's area, and the right pre-frontal area. These were found in varying combinations and degrees, depending on the individual. Although most deficits were found in the left hemisphere, some stutterers had them mainly on the right side and others had them bilaterally. After analyzing the data, the researchers came up with five "clusters" or subgroups of stutterers based on their neuropsychological profiles.

Other studies by researchers in Edmonton suggest that stutterers with severe neurological deficits are less successful in therapy programs than stutterers whose neuropsychological profiles are essentially normal. (Yeudall et al., 1993.)

What Is the Answer?

Although much is still unknown, we have identified a number of neurological factors that might promote stuttering by *increasing the difficulty of speech* or by *decreasing our control of interfering behavior*. In some cases, these factors may have been inherited. Alternatively, they could have resulted from conditions that affected the brain *in utero*, during childbirth, or thereafter.

However, these factors alone do not explain the development of stuttering behavior. As previously noted, the various deficiencies that have been mentioned by the researchers are not found in *all* stutterers, and they may also be found in persons who *don't* stutter.

For a more complete answer, we must look further. We must consider the ways in which these neurological factors may stimulate and interact with the Valsalva mechanism. In the next chapter, we shall see how a better understanding of the Valsalva mechanism might help us link together the pieces of this complicated puzzle.

General References

AMBROSE, N. G., COX, N. J., & YAIRI, E. The genetic basis of persistence and recovery in stuttering. *Journal of Speech, Language and Hearing Research,* 1997, 40, 567-80.

ANDREWS, G., CRAIG, A., FEYER, A., HODDINOTT, S., HOWIE, P., & NEILSON, M. Stuttering: a review of research findings and theories circa 1982. *Journal of Speech and Hearing Disorders,* 1983, 48, 226-246.

BLOODSTEIN, O. *A Handbook on Stuttering.* 5th ed. San Diego: Singular Publishing Group, 1995, pp. 100-102, 145-210.

BOBERG, E., EDITOR. *Neuropsychology of Stuttering.* Edmonton, Alberta: University of Alberta Press, 1993.

BORDEN, G. J., BAER, T., & KENNEY, M. K. Onset of voicing in stuttered and fluent utterances. *Journal of Speech and Hearing Research,* 1985, 28, 363-372.

BRAUN, A. R., VARGA, M., STAGER, S., SCHULZ, G., SELBIE, S., MAISOG, J. M., CARSON, R. E., & LUDLOW, C. L. Altered patterns of cerebral activity during speech and language production in developmental stuttering. *Brain,* 1997, 120, 761-784.

CIPOLOTTI, L., BISIACCHI, P. S., DENES, G., & GALLO, A. Acquired stuttering: a motor programming disorder? *Eur. Neurology,* 1988, 28, 321-325.

CONTURE, E. G., SCHWARTZ, H. D., & BREWER, D. W. Laryngeal behavior during stuttering: a further study. *Journal of Speech and Hearing Research,* 1985, 28, 233-240.

DE NIL, L. Some thoughts on the multidimensional nature of stuttering from a neurophysiological perspective. *Int'l Stuttering Awareness Day 1998 Online Conference, The Stuttering Home Page,* URL: www.

mankato.msus.edu/dept/comdis/isad/papers/denil.html.

DRAYNA, D., KILSHAW, J., & KELLY, J. The sex ratio in familial persistent stuttering. *Am. J. Human Genetics,* 1999, 65, 1473-75.

FARBER, S. *Identical Twins Reared Apart: A Reanalysis.* New York: Basic Books (1981).

FOUNDAS, A. L. Are the brains of people who stutter different? Stuttering Foundation of America website, URL: www.stuttersfa.org/Research/foundas.htm.

FOX, P. T., INGHAM, R. J., INGHAM, J. C., HIRSCH, T. B., DOWNS, J. H., MARTIN, C., JERABEK, P., GLASS, T., & LANCASTER, J. L. A PET study of the neural systems of stuttering. *Nature,* 1996, 382, 158-162.

FREEMAN, J., & USHIJIMA, T. Laryngeal muscle activity during stuttering. *Journal of Speech and Hearing Research,* 1978, 21, 538-561.

GOLDSMITH, M. F. Brain studies may alter long-held concepts about likely causes of some voice disorders. *Journal of American Medical Ass'n,* 1989, 261, 964-965.

HELM, N. A., BUTLER, R. B., & BENSON, D. F. Acquired stuttering. *Neurology,* 1978, 28, 1159-1165.

JONES, R. K. Observations on stammering after localized cerebral injury. *J. Neurology, Neurosurgery & Psychiatry,* 1966, 29, 192-195.

KEHOE, T. D. *Stuttering: Science, Therapy & Practice.* Boulder, CO: Casa Futura Technologies, 1999, pp. 70-73.

KENT, R. D. Facts about stuttering: neuropsychologic perspectives. *Journal of Speech and Hearing Disorders,* 1983, 48, 249-255.

MATEER, C. A. Neural bases of language. *Neuropsychology of Stuttering* (Boberg, ed., 1993), supra, 1-24.

MOORE, W. H. Pathophysiology of stuttering: cerebral activation differences in stutters vs. nonstutterers. *Research Needs in Stuttering: Roadblocks and Future Directions. ASHA Reports,* 1990, 18, 72-80.

MOORE, W. H. Hemispheric processing research. *Neuropsychology of Stuttering* (Boberg, ed.), supra, 39-53.

PAULS, D. L. A review of the evidence for genetic factors in stuttering. *Research Needs in Stuttering: Roadblocks and Future Directions. ASHA Reports,* 1990, 18, 34-38.

PERKINS, W., RUDAS, J., JOHNSON, L., & BELL, J. Stuttering: discoordination of phonation with articulation and respiration. *Journal of Speech and Hearing Research,* 1976, 19, 509-522.

PETERS, H. F. M. & BOVES, L. Coordination of aerodynamic and phonatory processes in fluent speech utterances of stutterers. *Journal of Speech and Hearing Research,* 1988, 31, 352-361.

REICH, A., TILL, J., & GOLDSMITH, H. Laryngeal and manual reaction times of stuttering and nonstuttering adults. *Journal of Speech and Hearing Research,* 1981, 24, 192-196.

ROSENFIELD, D. B., MILLER, S. D., & FELTOVICH, M. Brain damage causing stuttering. *Transactions of the American Neurological Ass'n,* 1980, 105, 181-183.

SHAPIRO, A. An electromyographic analysis of the fluent and dysfluent utterances of several types of stutterers. *Journal of Fluency Disorders,* 1980, 5, 203-231.

STARKWEATHER, C. W. Stuttering and laryngeal behavior: A review. *ASHA Monographs,* 1982, 21, 1-45.

STARKWEATHER, C. W. *Fluency and Stuttering,* 1987, supra, pp. 143, 159-165, 209-232.

VAN RIPER, C. *The Nature of Stuttering,* 2nd ed., 1982, supra, pp. 323-368.

WEBSTER, W. G. Hurried hands and tangled tongues. *Neuropsychology of Stuttering* (Boberg, ed.), supra, 73-127.

WYKE, B. The neurology of stammering. *Journal of Psychosomatic Research,* 1971, 15, 423-432.

WU, J. C., MAGUIRE, G., RILEY, G., FALLON, J., LACASSE, L., CHIN, S., KLEIN, E., TANG, C., CADWELL, S., & LOTTENBERG, S. A positron emission tomography [18F] deoxyglucose study of developmental stuttering. *Neuroreport,* 1995, 6, 501-505.

WU, J. C., MAGUIRE, G., RILEY, G., LEE, A., KEATOR, D., TANG, C., FALLON, J., & NAJAFI, A. Increased dopamine activity associated with stuttering. *Neuroreport,* 1997, 8, 767-770.

YAIRI, E., AMBROSE, N. G., & COX, N. J. Genetics of stuttering: a critical review. *Journal of Speech and Hearing Research,* 1996, 39, 771-84.

YEUDALL, L. T., MANZ, L., RIDENOUR, C., TANI, A., LIND, J., & FEDORA, O. Variability in the central nervous system of stutterers. *Neuropsychology of Stuttering* (Boberg, ed., 1993), supra, 129-163.

ZIMMERMANN, G. Articulatory behaviors associated with stuttering: a cinefluorographic analysis. *Journal of Speech and Hearing Research,* 1980a, 23, 108-121.

ZIMMERMANN, G. Stuttering: A disorder of movement. *Journal of Speech and Hearing Research,* 1980b, 23, 122-136.

ZIMMERMANN, G., SMITH, A, & HANLEY, J. Stuttering: In need of a unifying conceptual framework. *Journal of Speech and Hearing Research,* 1981, 24, 25-31.

CHAPTER 16.

The Brain and the Valsalva Mechanism

WHILE ORDINARY developmental stutterers don't exhibit the kind of brain damage found in acquired stutterers, speech scientists have reported a number of peculiarities in the way that their brains *function*. As discussed in the previous chapter, these findings don't solve the riddle of stuttering, but they do raise many new questions. For example:

• Is stuttering simply due to neurological weaknesses in the brain centers for speech, or is it caused by other forces that *block* an otherwise adequate speaking ability?

• Why are stutterers slower than nonstutterers in making voiced sounds, and why can they make a sound faster while *inhaling* than while exhaling?

• Are the abnormal muscle contractions in a stutterer's larynx due to reflexes that are triggered by changes in air pressure? If so, why would this happen only *some* of the time and not always during speech?

• Why do stutterers show unusually high levels of activity in the right hemisphere of the brain while speaking, and what relevance does this have to stuttering?

Much more research will be needed before these questions are finally answered. In the meantime, let's see if our Valsalva Hypothesis might suggest some logical explanations.

Weakness or Interference?

We have been told that stutterers are slow in starting phonation and poor in coordinating the movements of speech. Based on these and other deficiencies, some experts claim that stuttering is caused by a neurological weakness in our brains' ability to plan or coordinate the movements of speech.

But this can't be the whole story. As previously noted, there is considerable overlap between stutterers and non-stutterers: many stutterers are neurologically normal and many persons with neurological deficits don't stutter. Furthermore, it is not clear to what extent the neurological abnormalities are a *result* of stuttering.

In addition, we know that many developmental stutterers are capable of excellent speech when not blocked, and some are quite eloquent when acting out a role on stage. Indeed, our first-hand impression of stuttering is not that we *lack* the ability to speak, but that our ability is *blocked* by a force beyond our control.

What is the force behind these blocks? According to our hypothesis, it is the *Valsalva mechanism*. It is easy to see how this could throw off the timing and coordination of speech. When the Valsalva mechanism is activated, our body is neurologically programmed to perform a Valsalva maneuver — to build up air pressure, not to speak. Even when we seem to be fluent, there may still be some degree of interference, which could account for the slight delays that some researchers have detected in stutterers' fluent speech. Therefore, these symptoms would not necessarily indicate a defect in the speech mechanism.

Even when neurological weaknesses *do* exist, they are probably not enough, by themselves, to block speech in the typical developmental stutterer. However, by making speech more difficult, these weaknesses may increase a person's tendency to activate the Valsalva mechanism in an attempt to "force out" the words.

Therefore, neurological weakness may be one of many factors contributing to the anticipation of difficulty, which is Step 1 of the Valsalva-Stuttering Cycle. These weaknesses would not necessarily *compel* a person to stutter; they would simply increase the *likelihood* of stuttering.

Delays in Vocal Reaction Time

As discussed in the previous chapter, tests show that stutterers generally have slower reaction times than non-stutterers. This is particularly true in making a voiced sound in response to a signal. However, when the test subjects were asked to make a voiced sound while *inhaling,* the stutterer-nonstutterer difference in vocal reaction time was *cut in half.* Stutterers could make a sound faster while inhaling (called **inspiratory phonation**) than while exhaling (**expiratory phonation**), whereas nonstutterers were faster at the usual expiratory phonation. (Reich, et al., 1981.)

Why should stutterers' vocal delay be greater while exhaling than while inhaling? The Valsalva mechanism provides a possible answer.

During the tests involving expiratory phonation, the subjects were asked to inhale and to *hold their breath* while waiting for the signal. This was done by closing the larynx, causing a build up of air pressure. If the stutterer's Valsalva mechanism were overly active, the increased air pressure may have stimulated the larynx to continue the blockage of air, as in a Valsalva maneuver. In other words, the larynx would have been neurologically prepared to perform **effort closure** rather than phonation. As a result, the larynx may have needed additional time to readjust for phonation, thus prolonging the stutterer's vocal reaction time.

In contrast, you can't perform a Valsalva maneuver while you're *inhaling,* because then the lungs are expanding, sucking the air inward. Consequently, during the tests using inspiratory phonation, there would have been no increase in air pressure, no tendency to activate the Valsalva mechanism, and no interference with phonation. This explanation is consistent with reports that *stutterers speak more fluently while inhaling.*

Therefore, a significant part of an adult stutterer's vocal delay may be a neurological effect of the Valsalva mechanism.

Laryngeal Reflexes

Several researchers have linked stuttering to abnormal muscle contractions in the larynx that are inconsistent with phonation. These may include forceful closures of the airway, excessive muscular activity, and simultaneous contractions of opposing sets of muscles. Some experts have suggested that these may be involuntary reflexes that are stimulated by the increases in air pressure that occur during speech, and that the stutterer's brain may be deficient in its ability to suppress these reflexes.

However, we know that air pressure *always* increases during speech (for example, when we momentarily block airflow to articulate consonants), and yet developmental stutterers only stutter *some* of the time. Why should increases in air pressure trigger abnormal reflexes in some instances but not in others?

The Valsalva mechanism could account for this variability because it would be activated to a greater or lesser degree depending on our anticipation of difficulty. When the Valsalva mechanism is activated, the larynx is neurologically programmed to block the upper airway as part of a Valsalva maneuver. Certain laryngeal muscles will be ready to contract automatically in response to increased air pressure, in order to perform effort closure. The greater the air pressure during a Valsalva maneuver, the tighter the larynx closes to hold it in. The result would be a laryngeal block, such as those encountered on initial vowel sounds.

The Valsalva Hypothesis might also help to explain the other kinds of abnormal laryngeal behavior as well. It is possible that, while the stutterer is blocking in the mouth, the larynx is simply reacting to that struggle. However, the Valsalva mechanism might also contribute to laryngeal reflexes in other ways — either (1) by increasing the strength of reflexes, or (2) by interfering with the normal suppression of reflexes during speech.

The Valsalva maneuver is already known to strengthen certain reflexes. For example, I have seen doctors tell patients to do the hand-pulling exercise (described in Chapter 6) in order to enhance the knee-jerk reflex. Both Valsalva maneuvers and stuttering blocks have been shown to increase a neurological reaction known as the "H-reflex." (Lastovka, 1970.) Therefore, it is conceivable that activation of the Valsalva mechanism could heighten laryngeal reflex activity as well.

The second possibility is that Valsalva tuning may prevent the nervous system from suppressing the reflexes that interfere with speech. Neurological studies have shown that reflex activity (as measured by the H-reflex) is *lower* during fluent speech than when we are at rest. (Lastovka, 1970.) The "tuning down" of potentially disruptive reflexes may be a vital part of our preparation for speech. This process may get short-changed if we "tune up" the Valsalva mechanism instead.

Right Brain Involvement

As we have discussed in the previous chapter, the vast majority of people process speech almost entirely in the left hemisphere of the brain. In contrast, it has been reported that most stutterers tend to use the *right* hemisphere also. This condition is known as **bilateral speech**. In fact, the amount of speech activity in the right hemisphere seems to increase with the severity of stuttering and to decrease when stutterers become more fluent through therapy.

Why should it matter which side of the brain we use while talking? To begin with, the two hemispheres are usually not the same. Each is specialized to perform in a different way. The left hemisphere is superior in performing tasks that involve a rapid sequence of movements, such as speech. The right hemisphere, on the other hand, is slower, more "holistic" in its approach to tasks, and better at dealing with objects and spacial relationships than with words.

Experts have proposed a number of explanations relating stuttering to bilateral speech. Some say that the left hemisphere must be dominant in order to give proper timing and coordination to the muscles of speech.

Another theory is that the right hemisphere is more "emotional" than the left. Therefore, when the stutterer splits his speech processing between both sides of the brain, he increases the risk that his speech will be disrupted by emotional factors in the right hemisphere. One researcher has hypothesized that stutterers may have a "fragile" supplementary motor area that is disrupted by emotional overflow from the right hemisphere. (Webster, W.G., 1993.)

We shall now propose an additional answer: *that certain characteristics of the right hemisphere may increase a stutterer's tendency to activate the Valsalva mechanism when he anticipates difficulty in speaking.*

Because the right hemisphere is more adapted to dealing with *objects*, it may view words as being *things* that can be *forced out* with the same kind of physical effort that is assisted by a Valsalva maneuver. When the person feels that speech will be difficult, the right hemisphere may try to supply extra effort by activating the Valsalva mechanism.

It is hard to say which would have come first — the stutterer's use of the right hemisphere or his use of the Valsalva mechanism while speaking. Lateralization of brain functions develops gradually through childhood and may be influenced by learning. It is possible that stutterers have simply learned to process speech in ways that use the right brain's particular functions — such as viewing words as "things" rather than sequences of movement.[1] When, through therapy, a stutterer learns to approach speech as a time-related sequence of movements, he would be turning more to the special skills of the left hemisphere. The left side would then appear to be more dominant.

The Valsalva "Switch"

Even on the most fluent of days, we may feel that stuttering is "out there" somewhere, ready to pounce. We can be fluent at one moment and blocked the next. What can explain the swiftness with which our speech can change? Is there some kind of "switch" in the brain that quickly turns on the Valsalva mechanism?

Unfortunately, there hasn't been much research into how the brain triggers a Valsalva maneuver. Therefore, we can only suggest some broad possibilities while we wait for more definite answers.

Alternative nerve pathways. One way to explain the problem is in terms of the nerve pathways in a stutterer's brain. As we have previously discussed, the neurons in the brain connect with other neurons to form nerve pathways for various kinds of activity. These pathways may link up with other pathways to form complex circuits and networks. Some types of behavior may be served by multiple pathways.

It is possible that a stutterer's brain contains a number of different pathways for speech — including separate pathways for fluent speech and for stuttering. These pathways might follow different routes through the brain. Perhaps some go through the right hemisphere and others don't. Some might be linked to circuits that activate the Valsalva mechanism, while others aren't. Consequently, some of the pathways may lead to fluency, while others may lead to the Valsalva mechanism, resulting in excessive effort and force, interference with phonation, and other stuttering behavior.

When we anticipate difficulty in speaking, something in our brain may switch us from a fluent pathway to one connected to the Valsalva mechanism. The more we use such a pathway, the stronger and more habitual it becomes.

Where in the brain might this switch be located? Because stuttering is sensitive to stress and emotional factors, we might suspect areas deep inside the brain, including the **basal ganglia, thalamus**, and **hypothalamus**. The basal ganglia receive emotional inputs from the brain's **limbic system**. The basal ganglia are also involved both in turning on (through the thalamus) the appropriate parts of the cerebral cortex for speech and voluntary movement, and in turning off those bodily reflexes that might interfere with intended actions. The hypothalamus is already known for its ability to trigger rapid physiological changes in response to fear, as will be discussed later.

Brain chemistry. The Valsalva mechanism might also be activated by the release of chemicals in the brain. Various chemicals, including hormones and neurotransmitters, are already known to affect many bodily functions.

For example, we are all familiar with the sudden rush of adrenalin we feel when confronted with frightening circumstances. The heart pumps faster, our breathing is faster and deeper, our rectal muscles tighten, and many other physiological changes occur. This is the "fight or flight" response, which prepares our body to react quickly to threatening situations.

After years of research, scientists have found that this reaction is triggered by a chemical released by the brain's hypothalamus. This chemical travels to the pituitary gland, causing it to release a stress hormone into the bloodstream, which in turn stimulates the adrenal glands to pump adrenalin into the blood to stimulate the body to react to the emergency.

The Valsalva maneuver is such a common and instinctive behavior that it would not be surprising to find that it also had a chemical trigger. Such a chemical might be released when a person anticipates the need to use strenuous physical effort, or when the stutterer feels he must try hard to force out words. The discovery of such a chemical might lead to the development of other chemicals to counteract its effects, opening up new possibilities for an "anti-stuttering pill."

The Need for Research

Testing the Valsalva Hypothesis will require extensive research into the relationship between stuttering and the Valsalva mechanism — an area that has been virtually ignored by speech scientists. Because stuttering is not always accompanied by effort closure in the larynx (as would be expected in a typical Valsalva maneuver), researchers may have simply assumed that the Valsalva mechanism was not involved. They apparently overlooked the possible role of Valsalva tuning in causing forceful closures of the mouth, delays in phonation, and increases in reflex activity.

Up to now, the only published research I have found that even touched upon the Valsalva maneuver and stuttering was done in Czechoslovakia. (Lastovka, 1970, 1979a, 1979b.) These studies compared the effect of a Valsalva maneuver with that of a stuttering block on one type of neurological measurement, the "H-reflex." (While both increased this reflex, the effect of the stuttering block was somewhat greater, leading the researchers to speculate that emotional factors might also be involved.)

It would be helpful if researchers considered the Valsalva mechanism when designing future experiments. For example, studies of muscular activity during stuttering should include some of the significant laryngeal, abdominal, and rectal muscles associated with the Valsalva maneuver. The neurology of the Valsalva mechanism should also be fully explored.

Until researchers come up with a better explanation, the Valsalva Hypothesis provides a useful model of stuttering that fits together many of the scientific findings as well as the symptoms we personally experience.

Now that we have discussed the possible causes of stuttering, we shall examine, from the perspective of the Valsalva Hypothesis, certain conditions and techniques that seem to enhance fluency.

Note

See General References for complete citation.

1. Preliminary research at Vanderbilt University indicates that, between the ages of 3 and 5, non-stuttering children learn to process words as individual *sounds* (called "incremental processing"). In contrast, children who stutter continue to process words as a *whole* ("holistic processing"). Zackheim, 2003. These findings may lend support to our suspicion that people who stutter tend to treat words as "things" rather than as sequences of movement.

General References

BEATON, A. *Left Side, Right Side: A Review of Laterality Research.* New Haven: Yale University Press, 1985.

BOBERG, E., EDITOR. *Neuropsychology of Stuttering.* Edmonton, Alberta: University of Alberta Press, 1993.

LASTOVKA, M. The monosynaptic spinal cord reflex activity changes in stuttering. *Folia Phoniatrica,* 1970, 22, 129-138.

LASTOVKA, M. Influence of some psychopharmaca on the increase of the amplitude of electrically induced monosynaptic spinal cord reflex during the paroxysm of stuttering: I. effect of diazepam. *Folia Phoniatrica,* 1979, 31, 15-20.

LASTOVKA, M. Influence of some psychopharmaca on the increase of the amplitude of electrically induced monosynaptic spinal cord reflex during the paroxysm of stuttering: II. effect of chlorpromazine. *Folia Phoniatrica,* 1979, 31, 21-26.

NOBACK, C. R., STROMINGER, N.L., & DEMAREST, R. J. *The Human Nervous System: Introduction and Review.* 4th ed. New York: McGraw-Hill Book Co., 1991.

REICH, A., TILL, J., & GOLDSMITH, H. Laryngeal and manual reaction times of stuttering and nonstuttering adults. *Journal of Speech and Hearing Research,* 1981, 24, 192-196.

WEBSTER, W. G. Hurried hands and tangled tongues. *Neuropsychology of Stuttering* (Boberg, ed.), supra, 73-127.

WYKE, B. The neurology of stammering. *Journal of Psychosomatic Research,* 1971, 15, 423-432.

ZACKHEIM, C.T. Phonological priming in young children's picture naming: holistic versus incremental processing. (Presentation at Nat'l Stuttering Ass'n Conference, Nashville, TN, June 2003).

Part VI.

Fluency Enhancing Conditions

CHAPTER 17.

A New Perspective on Fluency Techniques

AMONG THE MOST INTRIGUING characteristics of developmental stuttering is its tendency to disappear, as if by magic, under certain conditions. Even severe stutterers are likely to be fluent:

- When singing;
- When reading in unison with someone else;
- When speaking in strict time to a metronome; or
- When silently mouthing their words.

Other conditions have a general tendency to increase fluency (although they might not be completely effective in every instance). These include talking to oneself, speaking very slowly, stretching out sounds, or using certain breathing techniques. In addition, some stutterers are quite eloquent when speaking with an assumed accent or acting out a role on stage.

Stuttering can also be reduced by changing the way a stutterer hears his voice — such as by feeding it back to him through earphones with a slight delay (**delayed auditory feedback**) or blocking it out by **masking**.

These are examples of **fluency enhancing conditions**. They do not "cure" stuttering. Once the special condition stops or the technique is not used, stuttering returns as usual. Therefore, the temporary improvement is sometimes called **artificial fluency**.

Why should such a wide variety of conditions tend to alleviate stuttering? What factors do they utilize that might help us control stuttering on a more permanent basis? Again, the Valsalva Hypothesis provides some promising answers.

Effects on the Valsalva-Stuttering Cycle

The wheel of stuttering is turned by a combination of psychological and physical factors that reinforce and perpetuate one another in a vicious circle. This is the **Valsalva-Stuttering Cycle**, previously described in Chapter 11. The fluency enhancing conditions can be explained by examining the ways in which they might disrupt various steps in this cycle.

Here are the six crucial steps in the stuttering cycle and the principal ways in which each of them might be defeated:

1. Anticipation of difficulty. Stuttering is usually preceded by our anticipation, either conscious or unconscious, that speech will be difficult. Based on past experience, we may expect trouble in saying a certain word or speaking in a particular situation (such as on the telephone). Or we may feel it's especially important to speak well under the circumstances. For whatever reason, we believe that extra effort is needed to get the words out.

This anticipation may be lessened by techniques that *simplify the mechanics of speech*, making speech seem easier. Our anxiety may also be relieved by conditions that *reduce the demand for good speech*, such as by making the words seem less important or by eliminating our need to make a good impression on the listener.

The expectation of difficulty depends not only on the words and speaking situations, but also on our perception of ourselves as stutterers. Therefore, fluency might be enhanced by circumstances that *improve one's self-image as a speaker*.

2. The urge to "try hard" by using physical effort. Once we feel the need to use extra effort in speaking, a crucial mistake may occur. For the reasons suggested in Chapter 16, the stutterer's brain may erroneously treat the words as if they were "things" that can be physically forced out by means of a Valsalva maneuver. Therefore, rather than processing speech in the normal way, the brain may activate the Valsalva mechanism to assist in this effort.

This tendency might be overcome by conditions that require us to *treat words as phonation and as a sequence of movements*, rather than as things to be forced out.

3. Valsalva tuning. Normally, the brain sends signals to the larynx within a fraction of a second before speech begins, neurologically "tuning" it for phonation. However, if the brain decides to force out the words with physical effort, it may "tune up" the Valsalva mechanism instead.

The larynx becomes the center of this confusion, because it is not only the voice box but also a key part of the Valsalva mechanism. It performs **effort closure** to block airflow during a Valsalva maneuver. Therefore, when the brain activates the Valsalva mechanism, it tunes the larynx for effort closure rather than phonation.

Valsalva tuning may be countered by methods that *focus attention on phonation* rather than force. If we mentally concentrate on using our voice, the brain will program the larynx for phonation rather than effort closure. The muscles for phonation will be ready to respond at the appropriate time, while the entire Valsalva mechanism will tend to relax.

4. Vocal delays and forceful closures. When the Valsalva mechanism is tuned up, both the larynx and mouth are prepared to block airflow in order to build up air pressure. As a result: (a) the larynx is not ready to phonate when it should, and (b) the larynx and mouth tend to close with excessive force, often in response to the increases in air pressure that occur during speech.

These effects might be reduced by techniques that either: (a) *prepare the larynx for phonation* rather than effort closure, or (b) *avoid abrupt increases in air pressure* that might trigger a Valsalva maneuver.

5. Avoidance behavior. When we sense that vocal delays or forceful closures are about to block our speech, we may resort to a wide variety of behaviors in an attempt to avoid, postpone, or break through the block. (These are described in Chapter 10.)

6. Reaction to stuttering. When we hear, or even *expect* to hear ourselves stutter, our original anticipation of difficulty is reinforced. Our ears are listening for the stuttering that we fear, and we are ready to respond with additional effort. We are taken right back to Step 1 and a repetition of the cycle.

One way to control this reaction is to *reduce the auditory monitoring of stuttering* — such as by preventing the stutterer from hearing himself. If we can't hear our stuttering, we may be less apt to struggle against it. Another approach would be to *increase our perception of the fluent aspects of speech*.

Now we shall examine the various fluency enhancing techniques to see how they might affect the steps in the stuttering cycle.

Speaking to Oneself

The most familiar of all fluency enhancing conditions is **speaking to oneself**, in the absence of a listener. In most instances, stuttering either disappears or is greatly diminished when the stutterer is alone. Of course, this is not always the case, especially when one is talking into a tape recorder or dictating machine.

Speaking alone affects Step 1 in the stuttering cycle by *reducing the demand for good speech*. Obviously, we don't need to make a good impression if no one is around to hear us. Therefore, we usually won't have as great an urge to "try hard." But this does not always guarantee fluency, because the presence of the listener is only one of many variable factors.

Silent or Whispered Speech

Stutterers are completely fluent when they mouth words silently (a technique called **lipped speech** or **silent articulation**). Obviously, this is not very useful in ordinary conversation, unless you are addressing someone who reads lips. Nevertheless, it shows that stutterers are perfectly capable of moving the lips and tongue — at least as long as the larynx is not involved.

Because there is no attempt to activate the larynx during lipped speech, there is no opportunity for confusion between phonation and effort closure. Therefore, Valsalva tuning does not occur.

Another explanation is that the absence of phonation *simplifies the mechanics of speech,* reducing the anticipation of difficulty (Step 1). One avoids the complex movements of the laryngeal muscles, the regulation of pitch and intonation, and the coordination of voice with airflow and articulation. Furthermore, the auditory monitoring of stuttering is eliminated, because you are silent.

During **whispering**, some disfluencies may occur, but the rate of stuttering is still much lower than in voiced speech. Although the larynx is used in whispering, it is on a much more limited basis. The larynx simply closes a little to cause some turbulence in the airflow passing through, in order to make the whispering sound. There is no need to repeatedly open, close, and adjust the vocal cords. Therefore, the mechanics of speech are greatly simplified, making speech easier.

Singing

Stutterers, as everyone knows, almost never stutter while **singing**. A part of the reason may be that music is processed in a different area of the brain than speech. Therefore, singing might employ a separate set of nerve pathways, which have not become entangled with Valsalva tuning and stuttering behavior.

In addition, *singing focuses our attention on phonation,* because the voice is what carries the melody. This would affect Step 3. While singing, we stretch out the vowel sounds and phonate almost constantly. As we listen to ourselves, we are not worried about stuttering, but rather we are concentrating on the pitch and musical quality of our voice. Therefore, our larynx is highly tuned for phonation instead of effort closure, and there is little chance that the Valsalva mechanism will interfere.

Slowed and Prolonged Speech

Slowed speech has long been recognized as a method of improving fluency. By this, we don't just mean pausing longer between words, but rather slowing down *during* the pronunciation of each word. For some stutterers, it may be necessary to speak *very* slowly, but there is almost always a point where fluency is achieved. (At least this is true in the therapist's office. In actual conversation the situation is a bit more complicated.)

The first impact that slowed speech may have on the Valsalva-Stuttering cycle is by *simplifying the mechanics of speech,* thereby decreasing the anticipation of difficulty (Step 1). When practicing the piano, it is easier to play a piece more slowly, because you have more time to figure out the notes and move your fingers. The same is true in speaking. You have more time to coordinate the necessary sequence of movements.

The muscles of the lips, tongue, and larynx have physical limitations on how fast they can move. According to some studies, these muscles move a bit slower in stutterers than in the average speaker. Therefore, stutterers may be attempting to talk at speeds beyond the capacity of their speech mechanism. This could increase the difficulty of speech and may create an urge to force out the words. Slowing down would remove this pressure by enabling the speech mechanism to work within its speed limits.

Even in the normal speaker, the lips and tongue don't have enough time to produce each sound separately. Consequently, there must be an overlap in movement, called **co-articulation**. For example, while the lips are forming one sound, the tongue may already be starting to make the next one.

Rapid speech increases the need for co-articulation, and therefore the complexity of speech. During slowed speech, we have more time to spread out the sounds and produce them individually. Therefore, speech is easier, and we have less temptation to force.

Slowed speech also *increases the emphasis on phonation,* affecting Step 3. Studies have shown that, when a person slows down his speech, he increases the proportion of time spent on the vowels as compared to the consonants.

A similar method of increasing fluency is **prolonged speech**, in which the stutterer stretches out syllables, especially at the beginning of phrases. Because the vowel sound is lengthened more than anything else, *phonation is emphasized.* Slowed and prolonged speech also help us spread out the pronunciation of words into their component parts, so we can properly treat them as a *sequence of movements*, rather than as things to be forced out as a single lump (Step 2).

Rhythmic Speech

Rhythm is another time-honored technique for creating artificial fluency. This method is simple and usually quite dramatic. Simply take a metronome, the kind used for practicing music. Start by setting it at a relatively slow speed (such as 60 beats per minute), and then talk in strict time to the rhythm. Each syllable should be spoken *exactly* on the downbeat. It — will — sound — some — thing — like — this. Very mechanical to be sure, but the chances are that you won't stutter. This fluency phenomenon is called the **metronome effect**.

After practicing a while, you can gradually speed up the metronome, first to 80 beats per minute, and then perhaps as high as 120. Even as speed increases, the fluency enhancing effect usually remains — as long as you say each syllable on the downbeat.

The effect of rhythm on fluency has led many people to assume that stuttering is caused by some kind of defect in the brain's timing mechanism. However, a leading authority, Marcel Wingate, has pointed out that rhythm also has a very definite effect on *phonation*. (Wingate, 1969.)

When a person says each syllable in strict time to a metronome, he tends to say the *loudest* part of the syllable at the same time as the *downbeat*. What is the loudest part of a syllable? Usually it is the beginning of the *vowel* sound — the very point when phonation is greatest.

As we speak in time with metronome, we will therefore be concentrating on *phonation* as we anticipate the downbeat. Consequently, the brain will neurologically tune the larynx for phonation rather than effort closure, and the Valsalva mechanism will be turned off (Step 3).

In addition, the metronome makes speech feel easier in a number of ways that would affect Step 1. It *simplifies the mechanics of speech*, both by slowing us down and by making all the syllables equal in timing and emphasis. Furthermore, it *reduces the demand for good speech* by providing an external force that seems to help us along. Some people might even call this a "crutch." Nevertheless, the more we rely on the metronome's beat, the less we will try to force the words out by using the Valsalva mechanism.

Choral Speaking and Shadowing

Stutterers are almost always fluent during **choral speaking** — that is, while reciting words in unison with someone else. They would have no trouble, for example, in a group recitation of the Pledge of Allegiance.

It's easy to speak along with a large group. There is no pressure to get the words out, because everybody else is doing it for you. Consequently, this situation *reduces the demand for good speech* (thereby affecting Step 1).

However, choral speaking can enhance fluency even without a group to back you up. All you need is *one* other person to read along with you — even if the other person is also a stutterer!

We have seen examples of this at our group meetings. Member A is at the lectern, blocking severely on some written material. When member B joins him in reading, A's stuttering usually disappears. As A continues to read, B gradually lowers his voice until it is barely audible. Nevertheless, A will continue to be fluent.

Speech scientists have confirmed the fluency effect of choral speaking in a variety of situations. In one experiment, the stutterer would face an audience all by himself, while reading in unison with a person who was speaking over a telephone. Even though the stutterer bore the entire burden of communicating the words to the audience, he still tended to be fluent. This effect occurs even when the stutterers read different material from one another.

Shadowing has a similar effect in reducing stuttering. In this technique, the stutterer has no written text, but instead plays "follow the leader." He listens to the speech of a fluent speaker and talks along with him, immediately echoing his words. You might try this sometime while listening to the radio.

Why do these conditions promote fluency? Hearing another voice may provide a *pattern of speech* for us to follow, thus making speech seem easier (Step 1). In some respects it may serve as a "crutch," like the metronome. But it may also remind us that speech is actually *phonation and a sequence of movements*. By following this pattern, our brain may be more likely to process speech in the proper way, rather than treating words as things to be forced out (Step 2).

Various Pressure-Reducing Techniques

There have been reports that stutterers speak more fluently while they are *inhaling* — a technique called **inspiratory speech**. I doubt it will ever catch on as fluency method, because it sounds terrible and is rough on the throat. Nevertheless, it does illustrate the relationship between stuttering and air pressure.

As discussed in Chapter 16, you can't do a Valsalva maneuver while inhaling, because the air is going in the wrong direction. The lungs are expanding, causing air pressure to drop. Therefore, inspiratory speech defeats Step 4(b) in the stuttering cycle by *reducing air pressure* rather than increasing it.

A number of less extreme speaking techniques may also affect Step 4(b) by *avoiding abrupt increases in air pressure* that might trigger a Valsalva maneuver. Here are brief descriptions of some common methods and how they work:

The airflow technique. Before speaking, the stutterer gently exhales a stream of air through his open larynx. Then he eases into his speech, prolonging the first word, while maintaining the airflow. Although other theories have been used to explain this method, its obvious effect is to keep the larynx open as much as possible, thereby avoiding the tendency to build up air pressure. It is essentially an anti-Valsalva strategy.

Easy onset. The stutterer begins his words and sounds in a soft and gradual manner. When beginning a vowel sound (as in "apple," for example), he starts with an open larynx and then *gradually* closes the vocal cords across the airflow until they start to vibrate. In contrast, "hard onset" would start by closing the larynx, building up air pressure slightly, and *then* releasing the vowel sound.

Light contacts. When forming consonants, the stutterer moves his lips and tongue as gently as possible, using a minimum amount of pressure. In this way, he tries to avoid physical effort and the forceful blockage of airflow.

These techniques have been incorporated into a number of speech therapy programs, which will be discussed in a later chapter. While they generally work well in the therapist's office, they are not always sufficient, in times of stress, to overcome the stutterer's overwhelming urge to force.

Other Fluency Enhancing Conditions

Many studies have shown that stuttering may temporarily disappear under conditions that change **auditory feedback** — that is, what the stutterer hears when he speaks. These findings have led some experts to speculate that stuttering is caused by a defect in the way we hear ourselves. In the next chapter we will point out the weaknesses of that theory and show how the fluency enhancing effects of masking, DAF, and other changes in auditory feedback are explained much better by the Valsalva Hypothesis.

We will also explore the reasons why some stutterers can be extremely fluent when speaking with an assumed accent or when acting out a role on stage.

General References

ANDREWS, G., CRAIG, A., FEYER, A., HODDINOTT, S., HOWIE, P., & NEILSON, M. Stuttering: a review of research findings and theories circa 1982. *Journal of Speech and Hearing Disorders,* 1983, 48, 226-246.

PERKINS, W., RUDAS, J., JOHNSON, L., & BELL, J. Stuttering: discoordination of phonation with articulation and respiration. *Journal of Speech and Hearing Research,* 1976, 19, 509-522.

ROSENFIELD, D. B. Stuttering. *Current Problems in Pediatrics,* 1982, 12, No. 8.

SCHWARTZ, M. *Stuttering Solved.* New York: McGraw-Hill Book Co., 1976.

STARKWEATHER, C. W. *Fluency and Stuttering.* Englewood Cliffs, N.J.: Prentice-Hall, 1987, 172, 188-196.

VAN RIPER, C. *The Nature of Stuttering.* 2nd ed. Englewood Cliffs, N.J.: Prentice-Hall, 1982, 418-426.

WINGATE, M. E. Sound and pattern in "artificial" fluency. *Journal of Speech and Hearing Research,* 1969, 12, 677-686.

CHAPTER 18.

The Effects of Hearing and Role Playing

IN THIS CHAPTER, we shall continue our discussion of "artificial fluency" by considering two additional categories of fluency enhancing conditions. The first group includes techniques that temporarily reduce stuttering by changing what we hear during speech, and the second deals with the effect of various kinds of role playing.

Hearing and Stuttering

Hearing the sound of our own voice is an important part of the speaking experience. This type of sensory information, called **auditory feedback**, enables us to judge the quality of our speech. While the various parts of our speech mechanism (the lips, tongue, larynx, respiratory muscles, etc.) are performing the physical movements of speech, our ears are listening for the final result — the *sound* of the words as they come from our mouth.

Normally, this information is used in a constructive way to improve the way we sound. For example, it may help us to regulate the loudness of our voice or to correct our pronunciation of words. But for a person locked in the grip of stuttering, auditory feedback may not always be so helpful. It may even tend to make stuttering worse.

The relationship between auditory feedback and stuttering has fascinated speech pathologists for many years. They have found that *stuttering can be reduced by removing auditory feedback or by changing it in various ways*. Three different approaches have been used to achieve this result:

• **Masking**, which prevents the stutterer from hearing himself talk;
• **Delayed auditory feedback** ("DAF"), which causes the stutterer to hear his voice with a slight delay; and
• **Enhanced vocal feedback**, which amplifies the vibrations of the vocal cords.

Why do these methods reduce stuttering, and what can we learn from them? As in the previous chapter, we shall approach this question from the viewpoint of the Valsalva Hypothesis. We shall see how each technique might disrupt various steps in the Valsalva-Stuttering Cycle, thereby reducing our tendency to activate the Valsalva mechanism during speech.

Masking

The first of these techniques, called **masking**, uses a loud noise to "mask" the sound of the stutterer's voice. In speech laboratories, this is often done by having the stutterer wear earphones that emit a constant "white noise" (which sounds something like the static on a radio when it's not tuned to a station). As the noise is increased to the point where the stutterer can't hear himself, stuttering usually diminishes.

For everyday use, the stutterer may wear a device called the **Edinburgh Masker**. Its main unit is a small box, about the size of a pack of cigarettes, which generates a loud buzzing sound while the stutterer is speaking. The noise is turned on and off by a small microphone strapped to the throat in front of the larynx. Plastic tubes carry the noise from the box to molded earpieces, which the stutterer wears in both ears.

While masking doesn't "cure" stuttering, it does demonstrate that most stutterers tend to be more fluent when auditory feedback is eliminated. This phenomenon is called the **masking effect**. It has long been known that stutterers are often more fluent when surrounded by loud noise (such as the sound of a waterfall or machinery). Similarly, studies have shown that *stuttering is relatively uncommon among people who are deaf.*

Effect on the Valsalva-Stuttering Cycle. In order to explain why the absence of auditory feedback helps fluency, we must first understand how the *presence* of auditory feedback might perpetuate *stuttering.*

Auditory feedback allows us not only to hear ourselves speak, but also to hear ourselves *stutter.* In this way, it may heighten our sensitivity to possible disfluencies, thereby contributing to our *anticipation that speech will be difficult* (Step 1 of the Cycle). Because of auditory feedback, we may feel pressure not only to impress other people with our speech, but also to sound good to ourselves.

Our anticipation of difficulty may then set into motion the subsequent steps of the cycle: the urge to "try hard" to force out the words by physical effort (Step 2); the neurological "tuning" of the Valsalva mechanism (Step 3); the resulting vocal delays and forceful closures of the mouth and larynx (Step 4); and the variety of behaviors we may adopt in an attempt to avoid, postpone, or break through the blocks (Step 5).

Masking may alleviate our anticipation of difficulty by *reducing the demand for good speech.* As previously mentioned, our own ears are among the "judges" we are trying to please. There would be little incentive for us to try hard to speak well, if we know we won't be able to hear ourselves anyway.

Auditory feedback may also have a significant impact on our *reaction to stuttering* (Step 6). Hearing our disfluencies may reinforce our original belief that speech would be difficult, leading us right back to Step 1 and a repetition of the cycle. Therefore, rather than helping us correct errors in our speech, auditory feedback may stimulate us to use even *more* force.

Masking would minimize this reaction by *reducing the auditory monitoring of stuttering.* If we can't hear ourselves talk, we can't hear ourselves stutter. Therefore, we are less likely to reinforce our belief that speech is difficult (Step 1), or to respond by doing all those things that make stuttering worse.

The effect of non-auditory feedback. Masking may also disrupt the Valsalva-Stuttering Cycle by changing the way that we perceive and process speech. According to our Valsalva Hypothesis, the stutterer's brain may erroneously treat words as if they were "things" that can be physically forced out of the body by means of a Valsalva maneuver (Step 2). Masking might help us avoid this tendency by creating a condition that encourages us to *treat words as a sequence of movements.*

Because masking eliminates auditory feedback, it forces us to rely exclusively upon various forms of *physical* feedback that come directly from the speech mechanism. One kind is **proprioceptive feedback**, which indicates the position of every part of our body in relation to every other part. This is what enables our finger to touch the tip of our nose while our eyes are closed. During speech, proprioceptive feedback tells us the exact location of our lips and tongue as we articulate.

We also use **tactile feedback**, involving the senses of touch and pressure. We can *feel* the vibration of the vocal cords, the contacts made by the lips and tongue, and the changes in air pressure as we form the words.

Whereas auditory feedback tells only about the *final product* (the sound of the words), the physical kinds of feedback deal with the *actual process* of speech. Whereas auditory feedback may permit us to treat words as "things," the non-auditory feedback helps us to experience words as *a series of physical movements.*

To some extent, these movements may be so habitual that they can be performed automatically, without our being aware of any feedback whatsoever. Each movement may trigger the next one, in a kind of preprogrammed sequence called **feed-forward**. Such a process might allow us to speak fluently when we are deprived of auditory feedback (and perhaps also on those occasions when we simply don't pay any attention to our speech).

Delayed Auditory Feedback

Another technique for enhancing fluency is **delayed auditory feedback** ("DAF"). Here we speak

Chapter 18 / The Effects of Hearing and Role Playing

into a microphone, which is connected to a device that delays the sound for a fraction of a second before feeding it back to us through earphones. Consequently, we don't hear our voice immediately, but must wait for a brief moment. The length of the delay is usually adjustable.

Although the time lag may be annoying, DAF has been effective in temporarily reducing stuttering. One explanation may be that DAF forces stutterers *to slow down their speech* and *to stretch out their words*. As a result, DAF may produce the fluency enhancing effects of **slowed speech** and **prolonged speech**, discussed in Chapter 17. By disrupting our usual auditory feedback, DAF may also force us to rely on **non-auditory feedback**, causing us to treat words as a sequence of movements rather than as "things" to be forced out.

When first discovered in the 1950's, DAF created a stir because of reports that it not only made stutterers fluent, but also *caused fluent people to "stutter."* Actually, the so-called "artificial stuttering" produced by DAF had nothing to do with real stuttering. When normal speakers prolong or repeat sounds under DAF, the prolongations occur in the *middle* of words, and the repetitions usually come at the *end*, like an echo — unlike real stuttering, in which disfluencies usually occur at the *beginning* of words.

DAF has recently enjoyed renewed popularity in the form of miniaturized electronic devices, such as the **SpeechEasy**, which fit in the ear canal like a hearing aid. The results are not perfect, and background noise often causes a problem.

Enhanced Vocal Feedback

A third approach is called **enhanced vocal feedback**. It changes the way we hear our speech by emphasizing the underlying sound of phonation. This could be done by placing a microphone against the Adam's apple, allowing us to hear the buzz of the vocal cords as they vibrate.

The same vibrations can also be heard through the bones of the neck and skull. They travel from the larynx to the inner ear by **bone conduction**. Therefore, it is possible to amplify these vibrations from a point close to the ear, without running a wire and microphone to the throat.

This method has been incorporated into a device called the **Fluency Master**, which resembles an over-the-ear hearing aid. It uses a tiny microphone pasted over the mastoid bone (directly behind the earlobe), to pick up the vibrations coming through the bones. The vibrations are amplified into a buzzing sound, which is heard through a molded earpiece.

You can experience a similar effect simply by covering the opening of one ear while you talk (a trick we learned from Dan Weiss of our local NSP group). Take the middle finger of your right hand, and lightly place the fleshy part of the fingertip over the opening of your right ear canal. (Be gentle, so as not to hurt your eardrum.)

Do you hear a loud undertone as you speak? That is sound of phonation, as carried by bone conduction. By covering your ear canal, you increase the resonance of bone conduction in your ear (a phenomenon called the **occlusion effect**), making it seem much louder than usual.

As you have noticed, one's voice sounds much different through bone conduction than it does through **air conduction** — the route with which we are more familiar. Through air conduction, we hear the sound of our speech after it has been shaped by articulation in the mouth. In contrast, the sound of bone conduction is *almost all phonation*. (This is why our voice sounds different to ourselves than it does on a tape recorder. The recorder hears only through air conduction, while we hear ourselves through bone conduction also.)

Enhanced auditory feedback has been reported to increase the fluency of many stutterers. We have seen evidence of this at our group meetings, when a few members experimented with both the Fluency Master and the occlusion effect. In some instances, the initial improvement in fluency was quite dramatic. Over the long run, the results were not as impressive (perhaps indicating that the original success was partly due to *distraction*, as discussed later in this chapter). Nevertheless, the technique continues to be helpful to some degree.

Enhanced vocal feedback may promote fluency because it tends to *focus our attention on phonation*. As discussed in Chapter 17, the more we concentrate on the vocal element of speech, the more our brain is encouraged to "tune" the larynx for phonation rather than for effort closure. This not only prepares our vocal cords to phonate more promptly, but also relaxes our Valsalva mechanism, reducing its tendency to interfere with speech.

In this way, enhanced vocal feedback may help to defeat Step 3 of the Valsalva-Stuttering Cycle.

Frequency Altered Feedback

Another variation on this theme is **frequency altered feedback** ("FAF"). As we speak, our voice is picked up by a microphone connected to a device that electronically changes the *frequency* of the sound and sends it back to us through earphones or an earpiece. We hear our words at the same *time* that we are speaking, but at a different *pitch*. The voice we hear may be anywhere from one-quarter of an octave to a full octave higher or lower than our own. As a result, the voice we hear sounds as if it is coming from *someone else*.

FAF has been found to have a significant fluency-enhancing effect during oral reading and some other speaking tasks (although it is less effective during monologue speaking tasks). The reason is not fully understood. Perhaps, as in the case of enhanced vocal feedback, the change in pitch *focuses our attention on phonation*. This may encourage the brain to tune the larynx for phonation rather than effort closure, thereby countering Step 3 in the Valsalva-Stuttering Cycle.

In addition, stutterers have reported that FAF makes them feel as if they are *speaking in unison with another person*. Therefore, it is possible that FAF may enhance fluency by creating the illusion of choral speaking. As discussed in the previous chapter, one reason why choral speaking promotes fluency may be that it *reduces the demand for good speech* (which would affect Step 1). This may also be true in the case of FAF, even though the "other speaker" is actually the stutterer himself!

FAF is currently employed in miniature electronic devices such as the **SpeechEasy**, which combines FAF with DAF.

Do Stutterers Have a Hearing Defect?

A number of speech pathologists, in attempting to explain the effects of auditory feedback techniques, have suggested that stuttering is a problem of *hearing* rather than of speaking. They have proposed that stutterers are defective in the way they process auditory feedback.

There are several different versions of this theory, none of which have been proven. One says that the stutterer's brain simply can't handle auditory feedback and needs masking to block it out. Another says that stutterers have some quirk that *delays* the processing of auditory feedback, creating an effect similar to DAF. But this seems inconsistent with the fact that DAF makes stutterers more *fluent*, and that the disfluencies caused by DAF are unlike real stuttering.

The story of the stapedius. Some experts have tried to connect stuttering to a tiny muscle in the middle ear. This muscle, the **stapedius**, regulates the loudness of sounds transmitted from the eardrum to the inner ear. It is also neurologically coordinated with the larynx, to protect the inner ear from the sound of our voice. When we intend to speak, the stapedius muscle contracts a fraction of a second *before* phonation begins.

The timing of these contractions is the same in stutterers as in normal speakers. (Shearer & Simmons, 1965.) When a person stutters, however, the activity of the stapedius does not simply parallel the vocal sound, as it does during fluent speech. It may also contract during the *blocks*, even though no sound is being produced. (Shearer, 1966.)

This behavior does *not* mean that the stapedius muscle causes stuttering, as is sometimes suggested. It is far more likely that the stapedius is simply *reacting* to signals being sent by the brain during the struggle to speak.

Weaknesses of the theories. Although the "hearing defect" theories stirred up considerable interest when first proposed, no one has yet been able to show that a specific hearing defect actually causes stuttering. Furthermore, the theories share some serious defects themselves. In particular:

- They are far too *narrow* in their application. They attempt to explain disfluencies strictly in terms of a few facts related to hearing, while ignoring many other aspects of stuttering. They create the impression that stuttering can be controlled *only* by masking or other auditory feedback techniques, when we know that this is not the case.
- They don't adequately explain the great *variability* of developmental stuttering. They simply assume that the defects are somehow aggravated by "stress" or "anxiety."
- They don't explain *silent blocks*, when no sound comes out of the stutterer's mouth at all. As we know, stuttering often begins *before* any auditory feedback can be heard.

In contrast, we have been able to explain *all* of the fluency techniques in terms of the Valsalva-Stuttering Cycle and the Valsalva Hypothesis. This approach provides explanations that are not only inherently logical, but also consistent with our previous explanations about the other aspects of stuttering.

In our view, there is nothing wrong with stutterers' ability to process auditory feedback. Instead, the problem may be in how we *use* the feedback. If we focus our attention on stuttering, auditory feedback may increase our urge to activate the Valsalva mechanism, making speech more difficult. On the other hand, if we listen for the music and resonance of our voice, auditory feedback can be a positive influence, guiding us toward improved phonation and fluency.

Distractions

Another view is that masking, DAF, and similar techniques are merely *distractions* — gimmicks that temporarily seem to improve fluency by diverting our attention away from stuttering. "Distractions" have gotten a bad name in the stuttering community, because they usually lose their effectiveness when the novelty wears off.

Even if distraction plays a role in the auditory feedback techniques, the results can still be explained in terms of the Valsalva-Stuttering Cycle. Anything that takes our mind off stuttering will tend to reduce both our anticipation of difficulty (Step 1) and our reaction to stuttering (Step 6).

The Fluency Effects of Role Playing

One of the colorful characters in Woody Allen's movie, *Broadway Danny Rose*, was a ventriloquist who stuttered — but whose *dummy* was fluent! I did not find this to be at all far-fetched, remembering how my own stuttering would disappear when I gave puppet shows back in elementary school. When I later took elocution lessons, I found I could stand before an audience and act out a role with perfect fluency.

Adopting an assumed accent also seemed to work magic. I remember a high school trip to Washington, D.C., where I achieved fluency by speaking with a Southern drawl — until my classmates finally told me to cut it out.

Similar experiences have been reported by many people who stutter. One member of our group became fluent when imitating JFK. John Harrison has told about his sudden fluency while portraying a Frenchman in a high school skit. (Harrison, 1999.) Some stutterers, such as James Earl Jones, have even become successful actors.

Although not every stutterer shares this experience to the same degree, there is no doubt that acting a role, imitating another person, and putting on an accent can often enhance one's fluency. While this phenomenon has led some observers to conclude that stuttering must be purely "psychological," it actually can be explained by the Valsalva-Stuttering Cycle.

As previously mentioned, our anticipation that speech will be difficult (Step 1) is based largely on *our perception of ourselves as stutterers*. We may view stuttering as somehow being an integral part of our personality. When we are really involved in acting, however, we set aside our old identity and let ourselves become another person. Consequently, this process may affect Step 1 by *changing our self-image as a speaker*.

Playing a character gives us license to "act out" and "let go," without being held responsible for what we say. This factor could also reduce our anticipation of difficulty, by relieving some of the ambivalence and self-restraint we might ordinarily feel in speaking situations.

When we "get into a role," we change the way we feel, move, and talk. We also breathe in a controlled way and vocalize with more phonation, in order to project our voice out to the audience. All these changes help us break away from our old behavior patterns connected with Steps 2, 3, and 4 of the Valsalva-Stuttering Cycle. Similar changes in speech also occur when we put on an accent.

Finally, the role-playing situations *change the way we hear ourselves*. We don't listen to our usual voice and expect to hear stuttering. Instead, we listen to "someone else" talking in a different way. We pay attention to the character's unusual accent or patterns of speech. We forget about stuttering as we get caught up in the performance. As a result, these situations may disrupt Step 6 of the cycle by changing how we react to our speech.

We have now completed our discussion of conditions that temporarily enhance fluency. In the next chapter, we shall turn our attention to therapy techniques aimed at controlling stuttering on a more permanent basis. We shall review the varied approaches to stuttering therapy, to see how they may affect the Valsalva-Stuttering Cycle and what might be done to increase their effectiveness.

General References

ARMSON, J., & STUART, A. Effect of extended exposure to frequency-altered feedback on stuttering during reading and monologue. *Journal of Speech, Language and Hearing Research,* 1998, 41, 479-490.

ANDREWS, G., CRAIG, A., FEYER, A., HODDINOTT, S., HOWIE, P., & NEILSON, M. Stuttering: a review of research findings and theories circa 1982. *Journal of Speech and Hearing Disorders,* 1983, 48, 226-246.

BLOODSTEIN, O. *A Handbook on Stuttering.* 5th ed. San Diego: Singular Publishing Group, 1995, pp. 90-92.

HARRISON, J. C. Why talking is easier when you are "being" someone else. *How To Conquer Your Fears of Speaking Before People.* 5th ed. Anaheim Hills, CA: Nat'l Stuttering Ass'n, 1999.

KEHOE, T. D. *Stuttering: Science, Therapy & Practice.* Boulder, CO: Casa Futura Technologies, 1999, pp. 179-181.

SHEARER, W. M. Speech: behavior of middle ear muscle during stuttering. *Science,* 1966, 152, 1280.

SHEARER, W. M. & SIMMONS, F. B. Middle ear activity during speech in normal speakers and stutterers. *Journal of Speech and Hearing Research,* 1965, 8, 203-207.

STARKWEATHER, C. W. *Fluency and Stuttering.* Englewood Cliffs, N.J.: Prentice-Hall, 1987, 183-188.

VAN RIPER, C. *The Nature of Stuttering.* 2nd ed. Englewood Cliffs, N.J.: Prentice-Hall, 1982, 369-395.

WEBSTER, R. L. *Fluency Master Procedures.* Hardy, VA: Epic Corp., 1989.

WEISS, D. M. Fluency enhancing systems . . . for free! *Letting Go,* Feb. 1992, 12, 2, 4-5.

WINGATE, M. E. Effect on stuttering of changes in audition. *Journal of Speech and Hearing Research,* 1970, 13, 861-873.

Part VII.

Stuttering Therapy

CHAPTER 19.

Stuttering Therapies Revisited

THE CONFUSION and controversies about stuttering are nowhere more apparent than in the realm of therapy. Through the centuries, hundreds of different methods have been used to treat people who stutter. These have included various forms of persuasion, punishment, surgery, mechanical devices, speech exercises, strange ways of speaking, relaxation, distraction, psychotherapy, drugs, attitude therapy, and behavior modification techniques. It is mind-boggling to think that a single ailment could have inspired such a diverse assortment of remedies.

We shall now explore this vast array of treatments, guided by the insights we have gained from the Valsalva Hypothesis. As we do so, it may be helpful to keep the following observations in mind:

- While some therapies are clearly more effective than others, almost *any* form of treatment will seem to benefit *someone* — at least temporarily.

- Although many therapies may seem totally unrelated to one another, or even contradictory in their approaches, virtually all of them can be explained in terms of their effect on the Valsalva-Stuttering Cycle. The success of any therapy may depend on its ability to disrupt one or more of the six steps in the Cycle (as discussed in Chapter 17), thereby reducing a stutterer's tendency to activate his Valsalva mechanism during speech.

- Thus far, no form of therapy has been completely successful in treating everyone. All have had limitations and drawbacks, and most patients have tended to relapse back into stuttering sooner or later.

- Many of these problems may be traced to *a failure to control the Valsalva mechanism in an adequate and efficient way*. Therapies have concentrated on speaking techniques and mental attitudes that have an indirect, "hit-or-miss" influence on the Valsalva mechanism. However, *no therapy has focused directly on the Valsalva mechanism itself.* As a result, some therapies may have hit the edges of the target, but none has scored a bull's eye.

In this chapter, we shall review some of the older methods of treating stuttering, which may help us to better understand today's therapies in their historical context.

The Power of Distraction

Distraction is an important element in many of the stuttering remedies that we will be discussing. People have repeatedly discovered that stuttering often disappears when some novelty is added to the speaking situation. Consequently, we will see that almost *any* method can bring temporary fluency — no matter how bizarre or illogical it might be. For example, a French physician once reported that he could control stuttering by pressing his thumb against his chin while speaking — clearly a method of distraction.

These gimmicks may seem to work magic, at least at first. In reality, they probably affect Step 1 in the Stuttering Cycle by diverting our attention away from our usual anticipation of difficulty or from other cues that trigger stuttering. Once the novelty wears off, stuttering usually returns. In many cases, the ineffective technique will remain as a habitual part of the stutterer's behavior, making his symptoms seem more bizarre than ever.

Persuasion and Suggestion

Since ancient times, many people have had the simplistic notion that stuttering is just a bad habit that can be overcome by exercising one's "will power." Therefore, stutterers have often been told such things as: "There's nothing wrong with you! You don't have to stutter like that!" In other words, "Snap out of it!"

Similar exhortations have found their way into stuttering therapy. Using a technique called **autosuggestion**, stutterers have repeated slogans aimed at convincing themselves not to stutter.

Perhaps the most dramatic form of this approach is **hypnosis**, which enjoyed some popularity during the 19th and early 20th centuries. Stutterers were put into hypnotic trances and given **post-hypnotic suggestions** that they would not stutter when they awoke. Back in the days when hypnosis was performed before audiences as entertainment, this was sometimes even done on stage. Stutterers would suddenly become fluent before your eyes — at least for the length of the performance. These demonstrations furthered the misconception that stuttering was all in one's mind, as well as creating the myth that it could be miraculously cured by hypnosis.

During my youth, I clung to the fantasy that my stuttering would someday be magically exorcised by means of hypnosis — a quick and easy cure that would require no responsibility on my part. In reality, however, post-hypnotic suggestions do not possess any special power. Consequently, the effects of hypnosis have been very unreliable and short-lived.

Although the power of suggestion can be a powerful tool for changing behavior, a negative suggestion such as "don't stutter" is likely to do more harm than good. The effort to use "will power" may encourage us to try hard by activating the Valsalva mechanism, making the tendency to stutter even worse.

A more beneficial approach would be the use of *positive* suggestions that emphasize, for example, the ease and fun of speaking regardless of fluency. These would affect Steps 1 and 2 of the Valsalva-Stuttering Cycle, by reducing our anticipation of difficulty and our urge to "try hard." Therefore, we would be less likely to activate the Valsalva mechanism in an attempt to force the words out.

The effect of positive suggestion is occasionally seen when a stutterer strongly believes in a particular therapist or kind of therapy. Similar phenomena may occur in the context of **faith healing** or other spiritual approaches. For example, if a stutterer believes that his speech is being assisted by some "higher power," he may feel less fearful of speaking situations and less dependent on force.

Unfortunately, positive suggestions usually have a hard time competing with the many negative memories about speech that we have accumulated over the years. At the first sign of relapse, a stutterer's faith may be shattered. Consequently, the power of suggestion is rarely enough to overcome stuttering all by itself.

Punishment

When persuasion fails, punishment has always been a popular way to try to change someone's behavior. Sadly, the same has been true in regard to stuttering. Throughout the ages, many stutterers have been subjected to corporal punishment, as their parents or teachers literally tried to beat the stuttering out of them. On rare occasions this kind of brutality may have worked. However, it is far more likely that such beatings would aggravate the fear of speech and stuttering, making the problem even worse.

Punishment has been a major component in many of the folk remedies that have been inflicted on stutterers. For example, stutterers have been forced to swallow goat feces, charred frog's tongues, raw eggs, mineral oil, and other unpleasant substances. They have been purged with cathartics, forced to chew garlic, and doused with freezing water.

Elements of punishment are also present in many forms of modern therapy. Patients are reprimanded or penalized for undesired behavior, be it stuttering or failing to use a particular speaking method. Some types of behavior therapy use punishment as a form of negative reinforcement. Stutterers have received various kinds of aversive stimuli, including bright lights, loud noises, and electric shocks.

Medical and Surgical Treatments

For hundreds of years, stuttering was viewed as a physical or nervous disorder, for which a motley assortment of medical treatments were suggested. Sometimes the remedies were relatively innocuous, such as rest cures, special diets, or the imbibing of warm wine to "loosen the tongue." Others were more unpleasant, such as the ingestion of nauseating potions, bloodletting, acupuncture, electric shocks, and the application of leeches to stutterers' lips.

But the most horrendous measures were reserved for stutterers' tongues. During ancient and medieval times, various physicians have advocated cauterization (burning) of the tongue, cutting its nerves, or cutting the frenum (the web under the tongue), on the theory that stutterers were "tongue-tied." The heyday of tongue mutilation came in 1841, when a Dr. Dieffenbach of Germany popularized the cutting of triangular wedges out of the base of the tongue. This operation was performed on hundreds of stutterers around the world, causing agony, infection, and even death, until it was mercifully discontinued.

Needless to say, such procedures had no therapeutic value whatsoever. If some stutterers initially seemed more fluent following their ordeal, it was probably because they were so distracted by pain that their anxieties about speech were temporarily forgotten.

Today, medical science has shifted its attention from the tongue to other areas, such as the larynx. For example, some researchers are using injections of **botulinum toxin** (similar to the botulism involved in food poisoning) to paralyze certain laryngeal muscles. At the NSP's 1993 convention, Dr. Christy Ludlow described such experiments conducted at the National Institutes of Health. The toxin was injected into stutterers' **thyro-arytenoid muscle** (which is used in closing the larynx). In some instances, a strong dose was used to paralyze the muscle completely on one side of the larynx. In other instances, lower doses were used to weaken the muscle on both sides.

For a few months after the injections, the subjects had a weak voice but generally didn't stutter as much. When the poison wore off, stuttering returned. One reason for this effect may be that *the paralysis prevented the larynx from blocking airflow, thereby reducing the possibility of a Valsalva maneuver.* (When I spoke to her after the presentation, Dr. Ludlow acknowledged that the injections to the thyro-arytenoid muscle would have prevented or substantially weakened the larynx's performance of a Valsalva maneuver.)

Drug Therapy

Less drastic remedies have involved the use of drugs. While it is natural for stutterers to dream of a pill that will bring complete and instant fluency, medical science has yet to find one. Thus far, medications have had only modest and inconsistent results in treating stuttering. While some stutterers are helped by certain drugs, others are not. In addition, there is the serious question of whether taking a drug is worth the long-term risk of side effects, when the same increase in fluency might be achieved by non-pharmaceutical methods.

Some stutterers have shown modest improvement while taking certain anti-psychotic drugs that block dopamine receptors in the brain. One such drug is **haloperidol** ("Haldol"), which is used to control behavior disorders. However, its side effects are so unpleasant and potentially severe that stutterers generally refuse to use it.

Another dopamine-blocking drug, **risperidone** (Risperdal), has been found to reduce the *severity*, but not the *frequency* of stuttering. (Maguire, et al., 1999.) Although risperidone is more tolerable than haloperidol, it still has potentially severe (and possibly fatal) side effects. Researchers are now investigating **olanzapine** (Zyprexa), another dopamine-blocker, which may have somewhat less severe side-effects, but still potential risks.

Some researchers believe that stuttering may be associated with excess dopamine uptake that may inhibit those parts of stutterer's brains that modulate speech. Theoretically, dopamine-blocking drugs might enable those portions of the brain to become more active, making speech production somewhat easier. If this is true, then the stutterer might feel less anticipation of difficulty (Step 1 in the Valsalva-Stuttering Cycle) and therefore less need to activate the Valsalva mechanism in an effort to force the words out.

To the extent that anxiety is a factor in stuttering, some stutterers have reportedly been helped somewhat by various combinations of anti-anxiety drugs, such as **alprazolam** (Xanax), and anti-depressants, such as **citalopram** (Celexa) and **clomipramine** (Anafranil). However, none of these drugs are considered a "cure" for stuttering, and all can have serious side-effects.

Researchers have also tested the effects of **verapamil** (a blood pressure medicine that controls muscle contractions), **bethanechol** (a remedy for constipation), and many other medications. Such drugs may work on the muscles or nervous system in various ways that may influence the Valsalva-Stuttering Cycle. The ideal drug might be one that specifically inhibited activation of the Valsalva mechanism. However, this approach has yet to be explored.

Speaking Exercises

One of the earliest approaches to stuttering therapy was based on the theory that stutterers had an underlying weakness in their speech mechanism. Stutterers were told to strengthen the muscles used for breathing, voice, and articulation by exercising them in various ways.

The most famous practitioner of this method was Demosthenes of ancient Greece. He strengthened his breathing by running up mountains with lead plates on his chest; he exercised his voice by shouting over the roar of the ocean; and he improved his articulation by learning to talk with pebbles in his mouth. These methods apparently helped Demosthenes, who went on to become the greatest orator in Athens. However, countless other stutterers who tried these methods have not been as successful.

Stuttering has also been viewed by authorities as a bad habit that could be broken by rigorous exercises in proper speech. This approach was widespread since at least the early 1800's. Stutterers were endlessly drilled in breathing techniques, vocal gymnastics, lip gymnastics, and proper articulation. The old books on stuttering therapy are filled with long lists of words, sentences, and passages that stutterers were required to recite for hours on end. Through this laborious process (called **massed practice**), stutterers were expected to overcome their habit of stuttering and to replace it with normal speech. When they still continued to stutter, the answer was, of course . . . *more practice!*

Similarly, many people who stuttered were once advised to take lessons in **elocution**. This is a method of public speaking that emphasizes clear and proper pronunciation, good vocal control, and dramatic gestures. I myself took elocution in my early teens. It greatly improved my skills in public speaking, enabling me to sound quite eloquent when reciting on stage. However, it did *not* cure my stuttering. Offstage, in normal conversations, I continued to block as badly as ever.

Exercises in speaking skills, such as elocution, acting, and public speaking, can nevertheless be helpful — as long as they are done in a positive, supportive way. On a neurological level, the practice may strengthen the nerve pathways for fluent speech. On a psychological level, stutterers may increase their experience, confidence, and pleasure in speaking. This may affect Step 1 in the Valsalva-Stuttering Cycle by reducing their anticipation of difficulty, thereby decreasing their urge to use the Valsalva mechanism to force out the words.

However, the strengthening of normal speech is only half the battle. Simply knowing how to speak well is generally not sufficient to control the forces that *block* speech. Other approaches must be found to accomplish that goal.

Mechanical Devices

Ever since the days of Demosthenes and his pebbles, people have been filling stutterers' mouths with all kinds of junk to keep them from stuttering. Some have been quite simple, like wads of cotton under the tongue or pieces of cork held between the upper and lower molars. Others have been more elaborate. Numerous contraptions were devised to keep the tongue in certain positions or to restrict its movement, including one with a sharp point to discourage the tongue from pressing too hard against the palate. Other devices featured tubes to keep the airway open and throat bands to compress the larynx.

If these appliances ever improved fluency, the effect was probably due to distraction rather than anything else. Consequently, they have long been abandoned as having no therapeutic value.

Nevertheless, we find that stutterers are wearing various kinds of "anti-stuttering" devices even today. Now, however, they take the form of sophisticated electronic gadgets. These include miniature electronic metronomes, such as the **Pacemaster**, worn like a hearing aid; the **Edinburgh Masker**, which produces a noise that prevents stutterers from hearing the sound of their voice; miniaturized delayed auditory feedback (DAF) devices, such as the **SpeechEasy**; the **Fluency Master**, which amplifies vocal vibrations; the **Vocal Feedback Device**, featuring an electronic vibrator on the throat; and frequency altered feedback ("FAF") devices, which cause stutterers to hear their voice at a different pitch (including the **SpeechEasy**, which combines FAF with DAF).

While these newer devices may act as distractors to some extent, they may also have other fluency enhancing effects, as previously discussed in Chapters 17 and 18.

Rhythm

The fluency enhancing effects of **rhythm** have already been discussed in Chapter 17. Its use in stuttering therapy is very old, dating back at least to the early 1800's. At that time, a French physician named Columbat devised a metronome-like device to help stutterers time their syllables to a steady beat.

Stutterers have since been taught many methods for adding rhythm to their speech, including foot-tapping, finger-tapping, and arm-swinging. One technique had the stutterer silently tap the fingers of his dominant hand in sequence, from the little finger to the index finger, and time each syllable accordingly. Another method required stutterers to trace an imaginary figure-eight, timing their breathing and speech to various points on the figure.

Rhythm dropped out of fashion during the first half of the twentieth century, only to re-emerge in the 1960's as a form of behavior therapy. It regained popularity with the introduction of miniature electronic metronomes, such as the "Pacemaster."

Rhythm has never been a totally satisfactory method, because the speech it produces sounds so artificial and mechanical that few stutterers will tolerate it. The therapist must gradually move the stutterer away from the strict one-syllable-per-beat rhythm in order to make the speech sound more natural. However, this often weakens the metronome effect, causing fluency to fall apart.

Novel Ways of Speaking

Many stutterers are more fluent when they deliberately talk with a strange or artificial pattern of speech. While this may be partly due to distraction, the enhanced fluency might also result from effects on various points in the Valsalva-Stuttering Cycle, as previously discussed in Chapter 17.

For well over a hundred years, speech therapies have conjured up fluency with such techniques as slow speech, prolonged or stretched speech, singing, whispering, speaking with a higher or lower than normal pitch, de-emphasizing consonants, emphasizing phonation, starting words with airflow or vowel sounds in order to keep the larynx open, and breathing in special ways.

A continuing drawback of these "artificial fluency" techniques is that they sound so unnatural that stutterers are reluctant to use them. Furthermore, they are difficult to mold into normal-sounding speech without losing their fluency-enhancing effects.

Although this approach to therapy was largely abandoned during the first half of the twentieth century, some of the old speaking methods were reborn in the guise of behavior therapy in the 1960's and 1970's. They currently form the backbone of many "fluency shaping" programs, which will be described in a later chapter.

Breath Control

Stutterers often display breathing irregularities during their struggle to speak. This fact has been known since ancient times. Exercises in abdominal breathing and other forms of breath control have long been a part of stuttering therapy.

Concentrating on proper breathing may serve as both a distraction and an aid to relaxation, thereby affecting Step 1 in the Valsalva-Stuttering Cycle. It may also discourage the activation of the Valsalva mechanism, by helping stutterers control their tendency to build up air pressure during speech.

Full breath. Some of the earliest advice to stutterers included the admonition to take a deep breath before speaking. Even today, a prominent "fluency shaping" program includes the taking of a "full breath" as one of its targets. The reason is obvious: an adequate air supply is needed to power one's speech.

However, the mere taking of a deep breath does not, by itself, guarantee fluency. On the contrary, this practice sometimes becomes part of the person's stuttering behavior. For example, some stutterers may take a deep gasp for breath and then *hold it in*, using their mouth or larynx to block the airflow. In these cases, the deep breath may do nothing more than provide additional air pressure for a Valsalva maneuver.

Costal breathing. A more extreme form of taking a deep breath is a technique called "**costal breathing**." Before speaking, the stutterer first releases residual air from the lungs and then takes a fast, full breath through the mouth, using rapid rib expansion and full diaphragmatic movement. Speech then begins aggressively at the top of the breath, without hesitation. The emphasis is on powering speech from deep down — without resorting to slow speech, easy onset, light contacts, or other fluency techniques that might cause one to "hold back" while speaking.

My impression is that the rapid intake of air and the exaggerated expansion of the rib cage and lungs during costal breathing may cause a stutterer to displace his "urge to try hard" onto the inhalation *before* speech, rather than focusing his effort on speech itself. Furthermore, the extreme effort used while inhaling may set up a condition in which the abdominal muscles then tend to relax more readily during exhalation. This muscular relation may have the incidental effect of relaxing the Valsalva mechanism and thereby reducing the likelihood that speech will be blocked.

While some people have found this technique helpful in controlling stuttering, costal breathing is nevertheless a strenuous, unnatural breathing pattern with distinct disadvantages. Among other things, it is hard to avoid making a loud gasping sound while inhaling, and using the technique during dinner conversation could be quite a challenge.

Airflow technique. Currently, there is a well-known therapy program that advocates the use of "**passive airflow**" as an aid to fluency. A gentle stream of air is released before easing into the first word. As will be discussed in a later chapter, such a strategy might serve to keep the airway open, thereby avoiding a build-up of air pressure that could trigger a Valsalva maneuver.

Relaxation

Because stuttering is usually accompanied by tension, many people have assumed that stutterers would become fluent by relaxing. Consequently, many therapies have employed relaxation techniques in the hope of reducing stutterers' tension while speaking.

These methods have included therapeutic bathing, sleep therapy, massage, prolonged periods of silence, hypnosis, auto-suggestion, visualization exercises, progressive relaxation, systematic desensitization, and biofeedback.

We shall defer our discussion of modern relaxation therapies to a later chapter. For now, we will simply point out that relaxation has had limited success in actual practice. The level of relaxation that stutterers enjoy in the clinician's office is almost impossible to maintain in the stressful environment of the real world. However, relaxation techniques might become more effective if they focused on specific parts of the body, such as the Valsalva mechanism.

Commercial "Stuttering Schools"

During the late nineteenth and early twentieth centuries, a number of commercial "stuttering schools" sprang up around the United States and elsewhere. They advertised heavily, charged high fees, and each promised a guaranteed "cure" for stuttering.

Stutterers came to live at these boarding schools for several months at a time. The first phase of treatment was usually a period of enforced silence, lasting several weeks. During this time, the students were instructed in relaxation and breathing exercises.

Then they were taught the school's secret "method" of fluency (which they were sworn not to reveal). These methods usually employed rhythm, sing-song speech, and similar tricks to produce temporary fluency. The students were drilled in these methods for weeks on end, given pep talks and slogans to build up their confidence in the method, and reprimanded when they failed to use the method diligently.

Although many students seemed fluent when they finished treatment, the great majority relapsed after a short time. By the 1930's, these schools and their methods had fallen into disrepute, as more "enlightened" psychological approaches came into fashion. However, with the advent of behavior therapies in the 1960's, many of the stuttering schools' old methods were given a new lease on life.

Modern Approaches to Therapy

The modern era of stuttering therapy began in the 1920's and 1930's, with the first serious attempts to approach the problem in a scientific way. At the University of Iowa, researchers developed radically new approaches based on stutterers' attitudes about their speech. Meanwhile, the writings of Sigmund Freud inspired efforts to treat stuttering through psychotherapy.

In the next chapter, we shall examine the strengths and shortcomings of these psychological approaches to therapy, which dominated the field until the behavior-modification revolution of the 1960's and 1970's.

General References

BLOODSTEIN, O. *A Handbook on Stuttering.* 5th ed. San Diego: Singular Publishing Group, 1995, pp. 407-452.
BRADY, J. P. Alprazolam, citalopram, and clomipramine for stuttering. *Stuttering Foundation of America website,* URL: www.stuttersfa.org/Research/drugther.htm.
BRADY, J. P. The pharmacology of stuttering: a critical review. *Am. J. Psychiatry,* 1991, 148, 1309-1316.
Burns, D. & Brady, J. P. Stuttering and speech disorders. *Psychiatric Clinics of North America,* 1978, 1, 335-348.
KEHOE, T. D. *Stuttering: Science, Therapy & Practice.* Boulder, CO: Casa Futura Technologies, 1999, pp. 74-78.
MAGUIRE, G. A., GOTTSCHALK, L. A., RILEY, G. D., FRANKLIN, D. L., BECHTEL, R. J., & ASHURST, J. Stuttering: neuropsychiatric features measured by content analysis of speech and the effect of risperidone on stuttering severity. *Compr. Psychiatry,* 1999, 4, 308-14.
VAN RIPER, C. *The Treatment of Stuttering.* Englewood Cliffs, N.J.: Prentice-Hall, 1973.
WEBSTER, R. L. *Fluency Master Procedures.* Hardy, VA: Epic Corp., 1989.
WESTBROOK, J. B. "Fluency-aids." *Letting Go,* Oct. 1992, 12, 10, pp. 1, 6-7.
WILLIAMS, J. D. 2,000 years of therapy. *Speak Easy Newsletter* (Paramus, NJ), Fall 1989, 9, 3, 4-5.
WILLIAMS, J. D. Use of the Edinburgh Masker. *Speaking Out* (Canada), May 1991, 8, 5, 7-9.
WINGATE, M. E. *Stuttering: Theory and Treatment.* New York: Irvington, 1976.

CHAPTER 20.

Psychological Approaches to Therapy

THE 1920's and 1930's saw fundamental changes in the nature of stuttering therapy. Earlier forms of treatment — such as elocution drills, rhythm, special speaking techniques, and other methods discussed in the previous chapter — fell into disfavor because of their failure to produce lasting cures. In their place arose a new generation of therapies, based on the premise that the key to stuttering did not lie in the mechanics of speech but rather in the stutterer's mind. The new therapies did not worry too much about the outward physical symptoms of stuttering. Instead, they focused their attention on various *psychological* factors that were thought to be at the root of stuttering behavior.

The psychological approaches began largely as a reaction to the quackery that had pervaded the field of stuttering therapy up to that time. Some of their early advocates were, in fact, stutterers who had been stung by the commercial "stuttering schools" — which had promised "cures" but produced only temporary fluency that quickly fell apart. In contrast to the superficiality of the earlier methods, the new approaches were supposedly based on more "enlightened" views of stuttering. They offered the hope that stutterers could permanently overcome their problem by changing from within.

These psychologically oriented therapies grew out of two separate schools of thought. The first approach, inspired by the psychoanalytic theories of Sigmund Freud and his followers, usually blamed stuttering on repressed emotions or conflicts, buried deep in the stutterer's unconscious mind. It tried to uncover and resolve these problems through various forms of psychotherapy. According to this theory, once the underlying conflicts were gone, the stuttering symptoms would disappear of their own accord.

The second approach was developed by early pioneers in stuttering research at the University of Iowa. It attempted to reduce the struggle and avoidance associated with stuttering by changing stutterers' attitudes about their speech.

Despite their good intentions, the psychological approaches ultimately created more confusion, frustration, and misunderstanding than ever before. To some extent, they were correct in recognizing that stuttering behavior can be greatly affected by unconscious thoughts and emotions. (Many of these factors have been previously discussed in Chapter 12.) However, in their single-minded pursuit of certain psychological aspects of stuttering, they usually tended to ignore the *physiological* side of the problem. Even worse, there were many psychotherapists (the Freudians in particular) who dogmatically insisted that stuttering was *solely* the result of emotional conflicts or other personality disorders, without any physiological component whatsoever.

In this regard, many of the psychological viewpoints suffered from the same kind of "tunnel vision" that has distorted other theories about stuttering. Therapies built on such narrow and shaky foundations provide little support for the person who stutters. As we shall see, they can even make matters worse.

Freudian Psychotherapy

Sigmund Freud profoundly influenced modern thought by showing how human behavior can be influenced by emotions, desires, fears, conflicts, and traumatic childhood experiences that have been repressed into the unconscious mind. For treating these deeply rooted problems, Freud developed an elaborate form of psychotherapy known as **psychoanalysis**.

In this intensive form of treatment, the patient lies on a couch and, guided by a specially trained analyst, embarks on an exhaustive search into his innermost thoughts, feelings, and memories. Among the techniques used in this process are **free association** (in which the patient reports whatever comes into his mind, allowing one thought to lead into another), analysis of the patient's dreams, and a phenomenon called **transference** (in which the patient develops feelings toward the analyst that are similar to those he originally felt toward his parents or other significant adults in his childhood). The analytic sessions may be as frequent as five times a week and may continue for several years.

Because of the tremendous cost of psychoanalysis, most psychotherapy has been more modest in scale. Typically, the patient meets with a psychiatrist or psychologist once a week and sits in a chair rather than lying on a couch. The therapist encourages the patient to talk about his problems, feelings, and memories, and helps him to resolve various issues as they come up.

It should be noted that Freud himself doubted that his psychoanalytic approach was appropriate for stuttering. Nevertheless, his followers came up with a number of theories (previously mentioned in Chapter 12) that attempted to explain stuttering in psychoanalytic terms.

Stuttering therefore found its way into textbooks on "abnormal psychology." Stutterers were branded as "neurotic," and their mothers were often blamed for causing them to have defective, stuttering personalities. These theories not only proved to be worthless in the treatment of stuttering, but they also caused indelible harm to stutterers and their families by inflicting shame, guilt, and social stigma.

Studies have shown that — regardless of its other benefits — psychotherapy is usually *not* an effective treatment for stuttering. The experience of the late Charles Van Riper, the well-known speech pathologist, is typical. After going through psychoanalysis, he found himself to be better adjusted, *but still stuttering*. I have heard similar stories from other persons who stutter.

I myself spent years in various forms of individual psychotherapy and more than a decade in psychoanalysis, plumbing the depths of my unconscious mind in search of the key to my stuttering. While I did gain some valuable insights into various emotional factors that may have increased my tendency to stutter, I never discovered any psychological "smoking gun" that would finally solve my problem.

The fact that psychotherapy rarely cured stuttering did not deter many devout Freudians. Instead of questioning the validity of their underlying theories, they interpreted their failures as merely demonstrating how deeply disturbed, and difficult to treat, stutterers really were. Thus, the fallacious view of stuttering as a "neurosis" was further compounded, leaving stutterers to feel more hopelessly crazy than ever.

It is possible that some stutterers in psychotherapy *did*, in fact, have emotional or personality problems that tended to *aggravate* their stuttering behavior (as previously discussed in Chapter 12). However, there was no justification for assuming that *all* stutterers had these problems, that these problems actually *caused* stuttering, or that they were the *only* factors involved. On the contrary, it seems more likely that the frustration of stuttering caused the emotional problems, rather than vice versa. Furthermore, as previously mentioned in this book, studies have shown that stutterers as a group are no more neurotic than the general population.

The limitations of Freudian psychotherapy can now be clearly understood in terms of the Valsalva-Stuttering Cycle. As we have seen, stuttering involves both physiological and psychological factors. Step 1 of the Valsalva-Stuttering Cycle begins with our anticipation that speech will be difficult. While emotional conflict may contribute to this perception (as previously discussed in Chapter 12), it is only one out of *many* factors that may do so. In addition, there are many other stresses or "cues" that may provoke stuttering in a given situation, even in the complete *absence* of emotional conflict. Freudian psychotherapy is therefore of limited value in alleviating stuttering, because it does not address these many other contributing factors.

Furthermore, because we cannot hope to eliminate *all* stress from speaking situations, an effective therapy program must help change the way we *react* to such stress — both mentally and physically. For example, it should help us to avoid the urge to "try hard" to force the words out, as if they were "things" (as described in Step 2 of the Valsalva-Stuttering Cycle). It should also include techniques aimed at controlling the Valsalva mechanism in a physical way, to keep it from interfering with speech (as described in Steps 3 and 4 of the Cycle).

Nevertheless, psychotherapy could be a useful adjunct to such a program, in helping to resolve emotional problems that may be aggravating a particular individual's stuttering or that may have resulted from years of disfluency. However, it must be based on a philosophy that recognizes the crucial importance of physiological mechanisms in stuttering behavior.

Varieties of Psychotherapy

Over the years, many psychotherapists have broken away from strict Freudian concepts in their attempts to explain and treat stuttering. The following is a brief assessment of only some of these variations.

Recognition of "repressed needs." One of my early experiences with psychotherapy introduced me to the rather simplistic notion that my stuttering was caused by my repression of unconscious needs and desires. Simply put, stuttering supposedly signified a conflict between what I was consciously *trying* to say and what I unconsciously really *wanted* to say. The proposed solution was to say only what I really wanted to, and to stop trying to say things that conflicted with my true desires.

As a naive high school student, I found this formulation to have great appeal. It gave me permission to stop trying to please others when I spoke, and for a while it *did* seem to improve my fluency. But the theory had a fundamental flaw.

If stuttering indicated conflict and fluency indicated harmony with my true desires, did this mean that I should say only what came fluently and avoid saying the things I stuttered on? (Like my name, for example?) Did this mean that I should avoid difficult speaking situations and confine my conversation to the kind of innocuous remarks that didn't cause me to block? And did it mean that I should refuse to answer when the teacher called on me in class? Obviously, this theory was neither accurate in explaining stuttering nor helpful in overcoming it. On the contrary, it was a prescription for disaster!

Releasing repressed anger. Another once-popular theory saw stuttering as a symptom of repressed anger. Some therapists therefore attempted to provoke stutterers to feel and express their anger. Often, this release of emotion was accompanied by temporary fluency.

This explanation seems to put the cart before the horse — since much of a stutterer's anger seems to be a *result* of his frustration over not being able to speak in the first place. Furthermore, the "anger" approach to fluency does not provide an appropriate long-term strategy, as I can again attest from personal experience.

During high school, I learned that I could be perfectly fluent when I let my anger loose. Therefore, I experimented with speaking in an angry tone of voice whenever I felt I was going to stutter. For a while this technique seemed to help, but I continually needed to increase my level of anger in order to maintain its effectiveness. Before long I had turned into a very surly, unpleasant person, whose angry fluency was rapidly alienating all his friends.

"Expectancy neurosis" therapy. Some psychotherapists do not see stuttering in terms of emotional conflicts or repressed needs, but rather as an **expectancy neurosis**, based on the stutterer's fixed belief that speech is difficult. According to this theory, it is simply the stutterer's *expectation* of difficulty that produces the stuttering behavior. Therefore, the goal of therapy is to disabuse the stutterer of this idea and to convince him that speech is actually easy.

In attempting to show the stutterer that he is capable of fluent speech, therapists have used some of the fluency enhancing conditions previously discussed in Chapter 17, such as unison reading and shadowing. The purpose was not to have the stutterer rely on these techniques permanently, but merely to change his mental expectations.

During the 1930's and 1940's, a technique called **breath-chewing** was used by Froeschels and others for this purpose. Stutterers were taught first to make vocal sounds while moving their jaws in large motions, as if speaking in some savage language. Then they would speak while making chewing motions, and then imagine they were chewing their breath while speaking.

These approaches to therapy might have an effect on Step 1 of the Valsalva-Stuttering Cycle, by reducing the stutterer's anticipation of difficulty and by changing his self-image as a speaker. However, it is hard to believe that stutterers' beliefs and behavior will be permanently changed by showing them a few gimmicks that conjure up temporary fluency. Most stutterers *already know* that they can be fluent some of the time!

What stutterers really need is a thorough understanding of why they stutter when they do and a way to control that behavior. Therefore, therapy should not only show that speech is easy; it must also explain exactly why stutterers make it so hard. As we have seen, the stutterer's basic misconception is his unconscious assumption that words can be forced out, as if they were "things," with the assistance of the Valsalva mechanism. In addition to dispelling this belief on a psychological level, therapy must deal with the stutterer's tendency to activate the Valsalva mechanism during speech on a *behavioral* level as well.

Cognitive therapy. This approach to psychotherapy (sometimes called **rational emotive behavior therapy**) is based on the theory that our feelings and behavior are influenced by the beliefs that we carry around in our heads. The therapist therefore helps the patient to identify the detrimental things he is telling himself, to recognize their falsity, and to replace them with improved beliefs through a process of rational thinking.

It is easy to see how this approach might be helpful in revising a stutterer's beliefs about the difficulty of speech, his attitudes about stuttering, and other harmful ideas. However, rational thinking alone is not sufficient to conquer stuttering. It must be integrated with a holistic approach that encompasses all of the steps in the Valsalva-Stuttering Cycle — both psychological and physical.

Attitude Therapy

The second school of thought, mentioned earlier in this chapter, emerged out of stuttering research done at the University of Iowa in the 1920's and 1930's. Originally the experiments were about cerebral dominance and changing the handedness of stutterers. However, those efforts were eventually abandoned in favor of various therapies based on the stutterer's attitudes and anxieties about speech.

This approach to treatment, commonly known as **attitude therapy,** was aimed at changing the stutterers' mental attitudes behind their stuttering behavior, such as their feelings and anticipations about speech and stuttering, their self-image as a speaker, their reactions to stuttering, etc. It was thought that many of these attitudes and feelings may have developed as a result of stuttering experiences. Although they were not the original causes of stuttering, they might nevertheless help to perpetuate stuttering behavior.

Therefore, stutterers were taught to look *objectively* at their stuttering, without all the fear and emotional involvement. They were encouraged to talk about stuttering in a free and open way. They were told not to look at stuttering as an external force that afflicts them, but rather as something that they themselves *do.*

This was the first type of stuttering therapy to which I was exposed, beginning back in high school. Once or twice a week, I would take a nauseating bus ride from my home town to a nearby city, where I was enrolled at the speech clinic of a major university. I remember sitting with a group of hang-dog, adolescent stutterers, telling a well-meaning young woman therapist how rotten we felt about stuttering. This went on for about a year, with nothing to show for it but several cases of bus-sickness. I was again placed in this type of therapy while I was in college, which at least did not require the bus ride.

Viewed in terms of the Valsalva-Stuttering Cycle, attitude therapy may affect Step 1 (anticipation of difficulty) and Step 6 (reaction to stuttering). However, it is difficult to change mental attitudes without backing up the exhortations with a clear understanding of the exact mechanisms involved in stuttering and teaching the stutterer specific ways to change his behavior to promote fluency. Therefore, attitude therapy should be integrated with other forms of therapy that effect changes in other steps of the Cycle as well.

Acceptance of stuttering. Some therapists carry attitude therapy to the point of saying that the goal of fluency is largely unattainable, and therefore the stutterer should simply learn to *accept* his stuttering and live with it. Rather than holding out false hopes, the therapist should teach the patient how to stutter openly in a more relaxed way.

Certainly, it is better to be a "happy stutterer" than to be frustrated, angry, withdrawn, and miserable. However, it is the rare stutterer who is satisfied with this approach. Most of us go to therapy for the specific purpose of reducing our stuttering — not to be told by the therapist, "Don't worry about it!"

Nevertheless, it is probably true that the road to fluency must begin with the acceptance of one's stuttering. It is difficult to understand and control stuttering while we are constantly hiding from it, denying its existence, or struggling against it.

Therefore, some therapies use an exercise called **voluntary stuttering**, in which the stutterer is assigned the difficult task of *stuttering on purpose* in various situations. One of the objectives is to reduce his fear of stuttering, so he will not react so fearfully to speaking situations. This technique will be discussed at greater length in the next chapter, in the context of behavior-oriented therapies.

Stuttering modification. Some practitioners of attitude therapy, including the eminent authority on stuttering, Charles Van Riper, eventually discovered that attitude change alone was not sufficient to control stuttering. People still continued to stutter, even when they no longer feared it. (This should not be surprising, because the fear of stuttering is only *one* aspect of Step 1 in the Cycle.)

Therefore, Van Riper expanded the scope of attitude therapy to include approaches aimed directly at the stuttering behavior itself. He devised various techniques to *modify* the stuttering symptoms and to help stutterers cope with their stuttering blocks.

In the next chapter, we will discuss these techniques in the context of behavior-oriented therapies, as well as exploring other forms of behavior modification techniques and "fluency shaping" programs.

General References

BLOODSTEIN, O. *A Handbook on Stuttering.* 5th ed. San Diego: Singular Publishing Group, 1995, pp. 407-452.
FREUND, H. *Psychopathology and the Problems of Stuttering.* Springfield, Ill.: Charles C. Thomas, 1966.
FROESCHELS, E. New viewpoints on stuttering. *Folia Phoniatrica,* 1961, 13, 187-201.
GLAUBER, I. P. Dynamic therapy for the stutterer. *Specialized Techniques in Psychotherapy.* New York: Grove Press, 1952, 207-238.
SHEEHAN, J. G. Theory and treatment of stuttering as an approach-avoidance conflict. *Stuttering Then and Now* (edited by Shames, G.H., & Rubin, H.). Columbus, OH: Charles E. Merrill Publishing Co., 1986, 187-200.
TRAVIS, L. E. The unspeakable feelings of people with special reference to stuttering. Emotional factors. *Stuttering Then and Now* (edited by Shames, G.H., & Rubin, H.). Columbus, OH: Charles E. Merrill Publishing Co., 1986, 93-122.
VAN RIPER, C. *The Treatment of Stuttering.* Englewood Cliffs, N.J.: Prentice-Hall, 1973.
WINGATE, M. E. *Stuttering: Theory and Treatment.* New York: Irvington, 1976.

CHAPTER 21.

Behavior-Oriented Therapies

IN CONTRAST to the "psychological" approaches to stuttering therapy discussed in the previous chapter, behavior-oriented therapies focus on what stutterers *do,* rather than what they think or feel. Such therapies pay less attention to the attitudes and emotions that affect stuttering, and concentrate more on the *physical* act of stuttering itself.

A wide variety of therapies may fall into this category. In this chapter, we shall look at several examples that have been popular in recent years. As usual, we shall analyze them from the viewpoint of the Valsalva Hypothesis, assessing their strengths and shortcomings in terms of their possible effect on the Valsalva-Stuttering Cycle.

Voluntary Stuttering

The first method we shall discuss grew out of research by Bryng Bryngelson and others at the University of Iowa in the 1930's. At that time, speech scientists were rejecting the older forms of treatment (such as rhythm, elocution drills, and unusual ways of speaking), on the grounds that their results were superficial and short-lived. Hoping to achieve better long-term results, Bryngelson tried an approach that was just the opposite of most therapies.

He called it **voluntary stuttering**. Instead of pressuring stutterers to speak fluently, this method required that they *stutter on purpose.* The stutterers were instructed to block intentionally on non-feared words — those on which no trouble was anticipated. This technique was based on the concept of **negative practice**. By stuttering intentionally, it was hoped that stutterers would be able to change the involuntary nature of their spasms into *voluntary* behavior that could be consciously controlled.

Originally, stutterers were told to observe their precise stuttering behavior in front of a mirror, and then duplicate the actual blocks when stuttering voluntarily. This proved to be a difficult task. Consequently, this approach was soon abandoned in favor of an easier, modified form of voluntary stuttering, called **voluntary controlled repetition** (or **"VCR"**). The stutterer was taught to repeat the beginnings of words in an easy, relaxed way, without using the excessive force characteristic of real stuttering. The stutterer was then assigned to go around in public, intentionally tuh-tuh-talking something like thuh-thuh-this.

Proposed benefits. Many speech pathologists have strongly recommended voluntary stuttering as a part of therapy. Several possible benefits have been suggested:

• *Acceptance of stuttering.* By stuttering openly, we relieve the pressure and anxiety that comes when we try to hide our stuttering or pretend that it doesn't exist. The benefits of this can be seen in terms of the Valsalva-Stuttering Cycle. Because we no longer feel the demand for perfect speech, we reduce our anticipation of difficulty (Step 1) and our urge to use physical effort in speaking (Step 2). Consequently, there may be less tendency to activate the Valsalva mechanism.

• *Avoidance reduction.* Voluntary stuttering forces us to confront our stuttering directly, rather than avoiding it. It short-circuits our tendency to use starters, circumlocutions, and other avoidance behaviors. This could have an impact on Step 5 of the Cycle (avoidance behaviors).

• *Desensitization.* Some experts believe that, by voluntarily stuttering in many different speaking situations, stutterers can reduce their fear of stuttering. To the extent that the fear of stuttering contributes to the anticipation of difficulty (Step 1 of the Cycle), this could ultimately result in less tension and greater fluency.

Drawbacks. Despite its highly touted benefits, voluntary stuttering has had serious limitations. Its first and biggest drawback is that most stutterers simply refuse to do it! I can easily understand why.

Although voluntary stuttering is supposed to help us confront our stuttering in an honest and open way, I have never felt very honest about using it. Voluntary controlled repetition doesn't sound or look like real stuttering, but rather like the pseudo-stuttering we sometimes hear when people try to mimic us. Listeners don't know what to make of it. Whereas a genuine block might arouse some degree of sympathy, the bogus quality of VCR is more likely to provoke nervous giggles or perplexed stares.

Furthermore, voluntary stuttering is rarely an adequate therapy by itself. Fear and avoidance of stuttering are only two of the many factors that contribute to the Valsalva-Stuttering Cycle. I would rather practice techniques that could accomplish the same objectives while at the same time promoting fluency in a more tangible way.

If one purpose of voluntary stuttering is to gain control over our spasms, then the behavior that we should target is not the tendency to repeat, but rather our tendency to activate the Valsalva mechanism during speech. Voluntary stuttering might be more effective if, instead of repeating the beginning sound of a word, we silently blocked on the word by doing a Valsalva maneuver — that is, by tightly closing the mouth or larynx and building up air pressure. We would then practice a method of releasing the block by relaxing certain parts of the Valsalva mechanism.

This exercise, called **voluntary Valsalva**, will be discussed in more detail in a subsequent chapter. It would not be as conspicuous as VCR, and yet would preserve many of the theoretical benefits attributed to voluntary stuttering. But most important, it would give the stutterer valuable practice in controlling and relaxing the Valsalva mechanism — the physiological key to stuttering behavior.

Stuttering Modification

Research at the University of Iowa spawned another influential approach to therapy, generally known as **stuttering modification**. Pioneered by the late Charles Van Riper (who was later at Western Michigan University), it sought to modify the *way* in which people stuttered, so that their symptoms would be less severe.

The stuttering modification therapies generally viewed stuttering as a collection of inappropriate learned behaviors involving the lips, tongue, jaw, larynx, and other parts of the speech mechanism. Stutterers were sometimes told to "freeze" the moment of stuttering in order to identify the symptoms peculiar to their individual patterns of stuttering. Various techniques were then used to help stutterers combat these symptoms.

One method was to replace the stutterer's tense struggles with a form of voluntary stuttering that utilized smooth prolongations of sounds. This type of speech is sometimes referred to as **fluent stuttering**.

Block Correction Techniques. Van Riper developed a number of techniques designed to help stutterers deal with their blocks more effectively. These consisted of three principal methods:

• *Pre-block correction.* Van Riper found that, before speaking, stutterers often held their mouths tensely in a fixed position, preparing to make the first sound. He referred to this initial position as a **preparatory set**. Van Riper believed that this rigid posture interfered with the relaxed movement needed for fluency. Therefore, he urged stutterers to adopt a preparatory set in which they began speaking with the mouth and jaw in a relaxed and neutral position. When saying the first sound, the stutterer was to keep moving *through* one articulatory position to the next, rather than becoming fixed in any one place. The stutterer was also supposed to begin airflow and voice immediately on the attempt to say the word.

• *Mid-block correction.* When stutterers found themselves stuck in the middle of a block, they were taught not to struggle, but rather to use a technique called **pull-out**. They were to finish the word with a smooth, controlled, gliding prolongation.

• *Post-block correction.* A third technique, called **cancellation**, was designed to correct a block *after* it was completed, on those occasions when the stutterer had not used the proper preparatory set or pull-out. After stuttering on a word, the stutterer was required to stop, think about what he had just done, and then say the word over again, this time in a more relaxed way. One of the purposes of this technique was to "cancel" the old way of stuttering and to replace it with "fluent stuttering."

Effects on the Valsalva-Stuttering Cycle. Some of Van Riper's techniques may indirectly affect the Valsalva-Stuttering Cycle in a number of beneficial ways. Because the speech objective is defined as "fluent stuttering" rather than normal fluency, the stutterer may feel *less demand for good speech*, thereby reducing his anticipation of difficulty (Step 1 of the Cycle).

The "preparatory set" technique, emphasizing constant movement *through* articulatory positions, may affect Step 2 of the Cycle (the urge to "try hard" by using physical effort). By reminding us that *words are a sequence of movements*, this technique may reduce our tendency to treat words as if they were "things" that could be physically forced out by means of a Valsalva maneuver. Finally, the techniques of "fluent stuttering" and "pull-out" both rely on the *prolongation of sounds.* Prolongation is a widely used fluency technique, whose effect on the Valsalva-Stuttering Cycle has been discussed in Chapter 17.

Problems. Stuttering modification has proven to be a difficult approach, requiring individualized therapy and intensive monitoring of one's speech. Numerous strategies must be learned in order to cope with the many varieties of stuttering behavior. Remembering and coordinating all these techniques during speech is a complicated task that may quickly fall apart in times of stress. Even when the techniques work as they should, the result is still not normal fluency — it is only *fluent stuttering.*

Stuttering modification therapies have had limited effectiveness because they fail to recognize the crucial role played by the Valsalva mechanism in blocking speech. Merely trying to modify behavior of the speech mechanism is not enough to control stuttering, as long as this underlying physiological cause remains unchecked.

Relaxation

The relaxation approach to therapy, which has a long history, gained renewed popularity in the 1920's and 1930's. It has continued to appear in updated reincarnations to this day.

The basic concept of relaxation therapy is simple. The therapist uses one of various techniques to put stutterers into a state of deep relaxation. Often this is done in a group setting, with several stutterers lying on mats, listening to a therapist speak in soothing tones. While they are perfectly relaxed, the therapist gradually instructs them to make sounds, form words, and speak sentences.

During relaxation, stutterers usually experience an immediate and dramatic decrease in stuttering. Unfortunately, it is a fragile fluency, which quickly crumbles when the stutterer returns to the outside world. The big challenge has been finding a way to reproduce the same level of relaxation and fluency in the stressful environment of ordinary speaking situations.

Relaxation techniques. Numerous methods have been used to induce relaxation in stutterers, of which only a few will be mentioned here. One example is **visualization therapy**, in which the stutterer is asked to imagine a peaceful scene described by the therapist.

Visualization is sometimes combined with a technique called **systematic desensitization**. After becoming totally relaxed, stutterers are told to imagine themselves in various speaking situations. They start with easy ones, like talking to a friend, and move to others that are increasingly difficult, like using the telephone or speaking before a group. These exercises are supposed to help stutterers control their tension when the *real* situation comes along. However, many stutterers have found that imagination and reality are worlds apart.

A more physical approach to relaxing the body is based on a technique called **progressive relaxation**, introduced by Edmund Jacobson in 1938. The patient is taught to relax various muscles groups, usually beginning with the toes and working all the way up. With each part of the body, the patient first tenses and then relaxes the muscles in question.

Nowadays, a person's control over muscle tension can be electronically enhanced by means of **electromyographic (EMG) biofeedback**. Electrodes, pasted to the skin, are used to measure muscle tension in a part of the body. This information is converted into an audible tone, which changes in pitch depending on the amount of tension. The patient can easily tell when he is relaxing, because the pitch gets lower. The object is to achieve maximum relaxation by making the pitch go as low as possible.

EMG biofeedback has been used in stuttering therapy to reduce tension in various muscles involved with speech. One researcher found that relaxation of the larynx and upper lip helped to reduce stuttering.

Evaluation of relaxation therapy. Relaxation may promote fluency by affecting the Valsalva-Stuttering Cycle on several levels. Psychologically, it may reduce our fear of speaking, and therefore our anticipation of difficulty (Step 1). It might actually make speech easier from a physical standpoint, because relaxed muscles are more responsive than those that are tense and stiff. Relaxation would reduce our urge to use physical effort in speaking (Step 2), as well as relaxing the Valsalva mechanism and preventing its activation (Step 3).

Unfortunately, stuttering therapies based on general relaxation of the entire body have a serious practical problem. It is difficult to keep oneself sufficiently relaxed, when assailed by the demands and stresses of everyday life. As Van Riper once said, "It's hard to be a limp rag in a steel world!"

However, fluency does not require relaxation of the entire body. The only muscles that really matter are those connected with the force behind stuttering — *the Valsalva mechanism*. It might be easier to maintain the relaxation needed for fluency if one simply concentrated on relaxing some of those muscles (for example, the abdominal and rectal muscles). Progressive relaxation or EMG biofeedback might help stutterers learn to do this, thereby enabling them to control the Valsalva mechanism during speech.

Fluency Training Programs

During the 1960's and 1970's, the face of stuttering therapy was again transformed — this time by new concepts borrowed from the growing field of behavior psychology. After much trial and error, there emerged a new batch of therapies that might be called **fluency training**. Although many different methods were used, most of these therapies followed a similar basic strategy:

• First, they would teach stutterers a peculiar method of speaking that promoted fluency. They relied heavily on fluency techniques of the past, such as slow speech, prolongation of sounds, continuous phonation, rhythm, or airflow. (The fluency enhancing effects of these and other methods have been discussed at length in previous chapters.) Stutterers were intensively drilled in the techniques until fluency was achieved. Often technological components were added, including delayed auditory feedback ("DAF") to slow the stutterer's speech, miniature metronomes worn in the ear to provide rhythm, or computerized monitoring of the stutterer's speech.

• After the particular speaking technique was mastered in an exaggerated form, it was molded into more natural sounding speech. This had to be done gradually, to prevent the loss of fluency.

• The final and most difficult step was training stutterers to use the new speaking method in their regular conversation. Modern behavior therapy techniques (including various forms of **operant conditioning**) were often employed to reinforce the use of fluent speech and to penalize stuttering. To help transfer the new skills to the outside world, stutterers would be assigned a "hierarchy" of speaking tasks, beginning with easy situations and working up to more difficult ones.

Fluency training was less dependent on individualized therapy than stuttering modification had been, because all patients could be taught the same basic speech technique regardless of their specific symptoms. Consequently, this approach lent itself to the development of standardized programs that could be administered to many stutterers at the same time.

Precision Fluency Shaping. Perhaps the most famous of these programs has been the **Precision Fluency Shaping Program** (now called "The Hollins Fluency System") sponsored by the Hollins Communications Research Institute in Roanoke, Virginia. Stutterers go for an intensive three-week program aimed at completely retraining their speech mechanism.

For the first week, stutterers are drilled in saying one-syllable words, spoken at a snail's pace of two seconds per syllable. Assisted by computers, they shape their speech in accordance with specified "targets." These have such names as "stretched syllable," "gentle onset," "reduced articulatory pressure," "full breath," "reduced air pressure," "slow change," "transfer," and "amplitude contour."

These targets incorporate numerous fluency enhancing techniques, whose effects on the Valsalva-Stuttering Cycle have already been discussed in previous chapters. Through massed practice, they are supposed to become habitual. However, it is doubtful that a person could remember them all when speaking under stress (for example, when responding to an angry boss).

The patients gradually move on to multi-syllable words and full sentences, until they master a technique called "slow normal speech." Then they are taken out to practice their skills in actual speaking situations.

Hollins is only one of many fluency training programs conducted throughout the United States, Canada, and other countries. While some are patterned closely after the Hollins model, others use their own training methods and emphasize different fluency enhancing techniques.

Phonation therapies. Some therapies emphasize phonation as a key to fluency. These include such techniques as **continuous phonation, legato speech, prosody,** and **vocal control therapy.** The general idea is to keep the larynx constantly vibrating, with little or no break in phonation between words. The monitoring of one's phonation can also be assisted by the "Vocal Feedback Device" or the "Fluency Master," previously described.

As discussed in Chapter 17, any method that emphasizes phonation may affect Step 3 of the Valsalva-Stuttering Cycle, by neurologically tuning the larynx for phonation rather than for a Valsalva maneuver.

Airflow therapy. Another highly publicized fluency program uses the **passive airflow technique,** popularized by Martin F. Schwartz. The stutterer is taught to exhale a gentle stream of air through the larynx before beginning to talk. This is to be done in a very relaxed way, without forcing the breath at all.

The stutterer then eases smoothly into speech, without interrupting the airflow, and stretches the first word or syllable. If stuttering still occurs, the stutterer then uses "low energy speech," talking softly, with as little effort and movement of the mouth as possible. Schwartz's program (which consists of a two-day seminar followed by a correspondence course) also includes exercises aimed at stress reduction and reinforcing the patient's use of these techniques.

According to Schwartz, his therapy is designed to combat the "physical cause of stuttering" — which he asserts is a locking of the vocal cords due to stress. While this theory has a certain simplistic appeal, it is contradicted by several studies showing that the vocal cords *don't* always lock during stuttering. (See Starkweather, 1982; Conture et al., 1985.) On the contrary, the point of blockage is often in the mouth rather than the larynx.

Airflow therapy can be explained much more cogently by the Valsalva-Stuttering Cycle. First, the airflow keeps the airway open, *avoiding a build-up of air pressure* that could trigger a Valsalva maneuver — as seen in Step 4(b) of the Cycle. Next, the stretching of the first syllable *emphasizes phonation*, affecting Step 3, as previously mentioned.

Shortcomings. Although modern fluency training programs may be more effective than therapies of the past, the astronomical "success rates" advertised by some programs should be taken with a grain of salt. None of these programs should be considered a miracle cure for stuttering. Many stutterers resist using the speaking techniques taught by these programs because they sound "unnatural." Others find the need for constant monitoring of one's speech to be an exhausting task. All too often, patients are fluent at the end of the program, but relapse after a few weeks or months.

These problems may be due, in part, to the fact that fluency techniques are only indirect and relatively inefficient ways of controlling the Valsalva mechanism. Even after completing a fluency program, stutterers will still be confronted with the Valsalva-Stuttering Cycle. When they anticipate difficulty in speaking (Step 1), they may feel an urge to "try hard" to use their new technique (Step 2). Not knowing any better, they may again succumb to their old tendency to activate the Valsalva mechanism, in an effort to help things along by "forcing" the words out (Step 3).

Once the Valsalva mechanism takes command of the mouth or larynx, all attempts to use fluency techniques may prove futile. Suddenly, the person may find himself back in the grip of stuttering — without any idea of how it happened!

General References

ANDREWS, G., CRAIG, A., FEYER, A., HODDINOTT, S., HOWIE, P., & NEILSON, M. Stuttering: a review of research findings and theories circa 1982. *Journal of Speech and Hearing Disorders,* 1983, 48, 226-246.

BLOODSTEIN, O. *A Handbook on Stuttering.* 5th ed. San Diego: Singular Publishing Group, 1995, pp. 407-452.

BOBERG, E. Relapse and outcome. *Stuttering Then and Now* (edited by Shames, G.H., & Rubin, H.). Columbus, OH: Charles E. Merrill Publishing Co., 1986, 501-513.

BOBERG, E., HOWIE, P., & WOODS, L. Maintenance of fluency: a review. *Stuttering Then and Now* (edited by Shames, G.H., & Rubin, H.). Columbus, OH: Charles E. Merrill Publishing Co., 1986, 489-500.

BURNS, D. & BRADY, J. P. Stuttering and speech disorders. *Psychiatric Clinics of North America,* 1978, 1, 335-348.

CARLISLE, J. A. *Tangled Tongue.* Reading, MA: Addison-Wesley Publishing Co., 1985.

CONTURE, E. G., SCHWARTZ, H. D., & BREWER, D. W. Laryngeal behavior during stuttering: a further study. *Journal of Speech and Hearing Research,* 1985, 28, 233-240.

JACOBSON, E. *Self-Operations Control.* Philadelphia: J.B. Lippincott Co., 1964.

LEE, B. S., MCGOUGH, W. E., & PEINS, M. A. A new method for stuttering therapy. *Folia Phoniatrica,* 1973, 25, 186-195.

PERKINS, W. H. Replacement of stuttering with normal speech: II: Clinical procedures. *Journal of Speech and Hearing Disorders,* 1973, 38, 295-303.

PERKINS, W. H. Do fluency controls ever promote automatic fluency? *American Journal of Speech-Language Pathology.* Jan. 1992.

PETERS, T. J., & GUITAR, B. *Stuttering: An Integrated Approach to Its Nature and Treatment.* Baltimore: Williams & Wilkins, 1991.

SCHWARTZ, M. *Stutter No More.* New York: Simon & Schuster, 1991.

SCHWARTZ, M., AND CARTER, G. *Stop Stuttering.* New York: Harper and Row, 1986.

SHAMES, G. H., AND FLORANCE, C. L. *Stutter-Free Speech: A Goal for Therapy.* Columbus, OH: Charles E. Merrill Publishing Co., 1980.

SHAMES, G. H., AND RUBIN, H., EDITORS. *Stuttering Then and Now.* Columbus, OH: Charles E. Merrill Publishing Co., 1986.

STARKWEATHER, C. W. Stuttering and laryngeal behavior: A review. *ASHA Monographs,* 1982, 21, 1-45.

VAN RIPER, C. *The Treatment of Stuttering.* Englewood Cliffs, N.J.: Prentice-Hall, 1973.

VAN RIPER, C. *Speech Correction: Principles and Methods.* 6th ed. Englewood Cliffs, N.J.: Prentice-Hall, 1978.

WEBSTER, R. L. Evolution of a target-based behavioral therapy for stuttering. Stuttering therapy from a technological point of view. *Stuttering Then and Now* (edited by Shames, G.H., & Rubin, H.). Columbus, OH: Charles E. Merrill Publishing Co., 1986, 397-414.

WEBSTER, R. L. *Precision Fluency Shaping (Vol. 1).* Roanoke, VA: Communications Development Corporation, 1974.

WEBSTER, R. L., & STOECKEL, C. M. *Precision Fluency Shaping Program: Speech Reconstruction for Stutterers.* Roanoke, VA: Communications Development Corporation, 1987.

WEINER, A. Vocal control therapy for stutterers: A trial program. *Journal of Fluency Disorders,* 1978, 3, 115-126.

WINGATE, M. E. *Stuttering: Theory and Treatment.* New York: Irvington, 1976.

WOLPE, J. Systematic desensitization based on relaxation. Behavior therapy of stuttering: deconditioning the emotional factor. Systematic desensitization. *Stuttering Then and Now* (edited by Shames, G.H., & Rubin, H.). Columbus, OH: Charles E. Merrill Publishing Co., 1986, 337-359.

CHAPTER 22.

Self-Help for Stuttering

PROFESSIONAL THERAPY is not the only avenue for controlling stuttering. Many persons who stutter have turned to various forms of self-help, either as an alternative or as a supplement to therapy. Some choose this route because they can't find therapy or can't afford it, or because the therapies they tried have failed. Others use self-help as a follow-up to therapy, a way of practicing and strengthening the fluency techniques they have learned.

Self-help should be clearly distinguished from the blind struggle to "stop stuttering" that many stutterers get locked into. When we speak of self-help, we mean a disciplined approach to improving one's fluency based on sound therapeutic principles. Therefore, self-help should begin by educating oneself about the nature of stuttering and ways of controlling it.

As we have seen, learning about stuttering can be quite confusing, due to the controversies over its causes and treatment. Hopefully, this book will make the task a little easier. Additional information can be obtained from the Stuttering Foundation of America (previously the Speech Foundation of America)[1], the National Stuttering Association (previously the National Stuttering Project)[2], the American Speech-Language-Hearing Association ("ASHA")[3], and other sources, including the Internet.[4]

In the next phase of self-help, the stutterer might practice speaking exercises and fluency techniques. These may be learned from self-help books or adopted from previous therapies with which the stutterer is familiar. Many stutterers practice by reading aloud. Some carry a small tape recorder to monitor their progress. A few may even experiment with their own methods of promoting fluency.

The precise forms of self-help chosen will depend on each individual and the resources available in his or her community. One of the most valuable strategies has been for stutterers to get involved in activities that increase their opportunity to talk and interact with other people. These may include, for example, participation in community projects, religious organizations, amateur theatricals, public speaking clubs, and — most important — self-help support groups in those localities where they are available. One's willingness to become *more active and outgoing*, despite one's stuttering, has brought greater long-term improvement in fluency than perhaps any other factor.

Self-Help vs. Therapy

As discussed in previous chapters, most people have found that no single therapy provides a total cure for stuttering. The early blush of fluency produced by some therapy programs may quickly fade in the harsh environment of the real world. A therapy that works wonders for one person may be a disaster for someone else. Many stutterers try several forms of therapy before they either find relief or give up on therapy altogether.

Stutterers' opinions of therapy will naturally depend on the degree of success they have had. A widely accepted rule-of-thumb is that, among all stutterers who undergo therapy:

• About one-third achieve substantial, long-term relief from stuttering;

• About one-third improve somewhat; and

- About one-third obtain no lasting benefit or end up worse than before.[5]

The most successful one-third will probably swear by whatever form of therapy brought them salvation. They may view therapy as being infinitely superior to self-help. The least fortunate ones, on the other hand, are likely to condemn all therapists as a bunch of charlatans. They may find self-help to be far more valuable (and economical) than the string of failed therapies that both dashed their hopes and depleted their bank accounts.

However, when we view professional therapy and self-help more objectively, it seems likely that *both* can be important to controlling stuttering. Used properly, they may complement and strengthen one another.

Even for stutterers in therapy, the spirit of self-help is crucially important to recovery. The control of stuttering is not something the therapist *gives* to us; rather, it is a skill that we ourselves must master through active participation. Speech therapists should be seen not as healers, but rather as *coaches*. They can instruct us in fluency skills, supervise our practice, point out our mistakes, and help us to correct them. But once we step outside the therapist's office, we're on our own. Therefore, we must learn to be our *own* therapists in order to maintain any gains in fluency that therapy confers.

Conversely, self-help is often a lot easier if the stutterer already has had a taste of therapy. Personal instruction and feedback from a skilled therapist is an experience that simply can't be duplicated by reading a book. Without professional guidance, stutterers may fail to recognize errors in technique or other self-defeating attitudes and behaviors that will impede their progress. Therefore, while self-help is essential to recovery, it's better if we don't do it entirely alone.

Apart from using a therapist, the stutterer might ask a sympathetic friend or relative to monitor his speech or otherwise assist in his exercises. Even more valuable help may be obtained from other persons who stutter, as found in self-help support groups.

Self-Help Support Groups

During the past few decades, self-help support groups have become a valuable resource for persons who stutter. In these groups, stutterers band together to help each other to help themselves. While the benefits of such an approach now seem obvious, the success of stuttering support groups has been a relatively recent development.

Many experts had previously doubted that stutterers had the inclination to form groups. It was generally assumed that stutterers did not like to talk to one another, that hearing other people stutter made them feel too uncomfortable. This seemed to explain why most attempts to start such groups fizzled after a short time.[6] A notable exception was the "Kingsley Club" (named after Charles Kingsley, an English author who stuttered), which was founded by lawyer-philanthropist J. Stanley Smith and which held meetings in Philadelphia and New York during the 1930's and 1940's. Another was the "Plus Club" in Sweden.

Stuttering groups did not gain a foothold until the late 1960's or 1970's — about the same time that other kinds of support groups became popular throughout our society. The National Council for Adult Stutterers began in 1966[7], the National Council on Stuttering[8] was founded in 1974 and the National Stuttering Project — now known as the National Stuttering Association ("NSA") — was born in 1977.[9] Other groups now include Speak Easy International[10] in the United States, Speak Easy[11] in Canada, the Canadian Association for People who Stutter ("CAPS"),[12] and numerous similar groups in many countries.[13] The movement has grown to world-wide dimensions, with the creation of the International Stuttering Association[14] in 1995 and the periodic holding of international conventions for people who stutter.

Support groups now meet regularly in many localities. These groups help stutterers build self-confidence and self-respect, as well as providing a bridge between therapy and ordinary speaking situations. At the meetings, the group members can discuss their thoughts, feelings, and experiences about stuttering; gain experience speaking before a group in a supportive environment; practice fluency techniques they may be trying out; and socialize with people who have a common bond. The cost of joining such groups is usually minimal.

Some groups are intended to serve as extensions of particular forms of therapy. In some groups, for example, members practice the targets they have learned in the Precision Fluency Shaping

Program. Other groups are centered around the air-flow technique. However, most groups (including the NSA) are not based on any fluency method, but try instead to make people feel more comfortable with their stuttering.

Many of the groups publish newsletters, which provide information about stuttering research and therapy and permit stutterers to share their experiences and ideas with one another. Other activities may include educating the public and combatting prejudice and discrimination against persons who stutter. Organizations such as the NSA periodically hold regional workshops and national conventions.

In terms of the Valsalva-Stuttering Cycle, participation in support groups may reduce the anticipation of difficulty in speaking, thereby affecting Step 1. The groups provide moral support, showing the stutterer that he or she is not alone. They help stutterers to increase self-esteem, to view stuttering more objectively, and to feel less ashamed. These changes in attitude may also have a beneficial effect on Step 6 (the reaction to stuttering).

The Support Group Experience

My own experience with support groups, based on several years of involvement with the NSA and contact with a few other groups, has been overwhelmingly positive. My only regret is that such groups were not available when I was growing up.

Before I joined the NSA, stuttering was not something I could talk about. I thought it was too shameful, too embarrassing. I did not even feel comfortable discussing the subject with other stutterers I met. I painfully remember the group therapy sessions I attended at a university's speech department. Being there made me feel like a defective misfit. Seeing someone else stutter only made me feel worse about myself.

Our relationship to speech pathologists and therapists is based on the idea that we are abnormal, that there is something *wrong* with us. In contrast, self-help groups like the NSA offer a totally different experience. Together, we are a lively, optimistic bunch. The meetings of our local group are filled with laughter and good cheer. Our getting together affirms what is *right* with us. Rather than feeling like "patients" who have come to a therapist to be "cured," we are our *own* therapists. We are in control. We accept responsibility for our own speech and do what we can to improve it.

In the NSA, stuttering is not seen as shameful, but rather as an ordeal that we have shared in common, which has initiated us into a fraternity. Stuttering has touched our egos so deeply and shaped our lives so pervasively, that we who have experienced it are bonded in kinship. To other members of the NSA, we are like brothers and sisters. By recognizing and affirming one another, we each affirm ourselves. In this affirmation lies self-acceptance and the pathway to growth.

Limitations of Support Groups

Perhaps the biggest problem with stuttering support groups is that many areas don't have them and, in most localities where they exist, they are sadly under-utilized. A group's success depends on dynamic and dedicated leadership, as well as a sufficiently large community of stutterers to participate in its meetings and other activities.

These groups often begin with a flurry of publicity, with many stutterers attending the first few meetings, mainly out of curiosity. For various reasons, a majority of the visitors quickly drop out, leaving a relatively small core of members who keep the group going for a while. As these people gradually lose interest, attendance further dwindles. Therefore, unless a group receives a continuous infusion of new blood, it will languish and die. Consequently, support groups stand a better chance of survival in large urban areas, where they can draw upon a virtually inexhaustible pool of stutterers.

People who come to support groups expecting a magic cure are bound to go away disappointed. As we have seen, there is no easy solution to stuttering. Those demanding a quick fix will miss the real advantages the groups have to offer.

Stuttering support groups are generally not in a position to do much speech therapy, except on a relatively superficial level. Furthermore, they usually lack the kind of therapeutic or inspirational program that holds together many other self-help organizations, such as Alcoholics Anonymous or Weight Watchers. This may be due, in part, to disagreements among stutterers about the role that support groups should play. Some members would like meetings to include practice in fluency techniques; others simply want an opportunity to speak or to ventilate their feelings. Some believe that a group's purpose should be to promote fluency; others believe it should be to help members live with their stuttering.

At least one group has tried to duplicate the success of Alcoholics Anonymous by adapting AA's famous "12-Step Program." [15] However, this approach forces us to treat stuttering as if it were an addiction like alcoholism and drug dependency — which it obviously is not. No matter how inspirational or otherwise helpful the 12 Steps may be, they are no substitute for understanding the true nature of our problem. It would be far better to tailor a program specifically for stuttering than to squeeze stuttering into a mold it does not fit.

Ideally, stuttering support groups should develop a comprehensive approach that not only inspires self-respect, but also provides members with a theoretical basis for understanding stuttering and practical guidelines for controlling it.

What Self-Help Therapy Program?

Regardless of whether one pursues professional therapy, self-help, or a combination of both, one's success at controlling stuttering will depend largely on the therapeutic methods that are actually employed. As discussed in the preceding chapters, all the existing therapies have limitations and shortcomings. None of them focuses sufficiently on controlling the Valsalva mechanism — which may be the principal force behind stuttering behavior. While many therapies affect *some* steps of the Valsalva-Stuttering Cycle, they do so in an indirect and relatively inefficient way.

According to our hypothesis, therapy would be more effective if it directly attacked *all six points of the Valsalva-Stuttering Cycle*. In the next part of this book, we shall take a first step toward developing such a program. We shall suggest an experimental approach for improving fluency, which will employ both physical and psychological techniques aimed at controlling the Valsalva mechanism and breaking the Valsalva-Stuttering cycle.

Notes

See Bibliography for complete citation of references.

1. For a list of publications, write to the Stuttering Foundation of America, P.O. Box 11749, 3100 Walnut Grove Road, No. 603, Memphis, TN 38111-0749. Website: www.stuttersfa.org. Of particular interest is Fraser, M., *Self-Therapy for the Stutterer*, Publication No. 12 (7th ed., 1990).

2. Write or call the National Stuttering Association, 407119 W. 40th Street, 14th Floor, New York, NY 10018; telephone 1-800-WE STUTTER. Website: www.WeStutter.org.

3. American Speech-Language-Hearing Association, 10801 Rockville Pike, Rockville, MD 20852; telephone: (301) 897-5700 or 1-800-638-8255. Website: www.asha.org.

4. A good place to start on the Internet is The Stuttering Home Page, maintained by Judith Kuster, an associate professor at Minnesota State University, Mankato, in consultation with John C. Harrison. It can be found on the web at www.stutteringhomepage.com or http://mankato.msus.edu/~stutter.

5. Murray, F.P., Commentary, *The Speak Easy Newsletter,* Spring 1992, 12,1, p. 6.

6. Van Riper, C., *The Treatment of Stuttering*, 168-170.

7. See Van Riper, C., *The Treatment of Stuttering*, p. 169.

8. The National Council on Stuttering, 1200 W. Harrison Street, Suite 2010, Chicago, IL 60607.

9. Sugarman, M., NSP going strong: a little history — Part I, *Letting Go,* July 1990, 3-4; — Part II, *Letting Go,* Aug. 1990, 5-6.

10. Speak Easy International Foundation, Inc., 233 Concord Drive, Paramus, NJ 07652.

11. Speak Easy, Inc., 95 Evergreen Ave., Saint John, NB, Canada E2N 1H4. URL: www.speakeasycanada.com.

12. Canadian Association for People Who Stutter ("CAPS"), P.O. Box 444, Branch NDG, Montreal QC H4A 3P8, Canada. Website: www.webcon.net/~caps/.

13. See Appendix B for a partial list of stuttering self-help organizations in the United States, Canada, and other countries.

14. International Stuttering Association website: www.stutterisa.org.

15. Compulsive Stutterers Anonymous, Box 1406, Park Ridge, IL 60068. See Reed, 1990.

Part VIII.

Breaking the Valsalva-Stuttering Cycle

CHAPTER 23.

The Principles of Valsalva Control

NOW THAT WE HAVE PIECED together a detailed picture of stuttering based on the Valsalva Hypothesis, we are ready to tackle the ultimate question: How can this new understanding help us to *control* stuttering?

In our view, most stuttering is not caused by any lack of *ability* to speak fluently, but rather by an *interference* with that ability by the Valsalva mechanism — the bodily mechanism for exerting force. We have seen how this tendency is perpetuated by various psychological and physiological factors that make up the Valsalva-Stuttering Cycle. After years of stuttering, these behaviors become deeply rooted in the nerve pathways of the brain, making them extremely difficult to change.

This part of the book will lay out a comprehensive game plan to improve fluency by controlling the Valsalva mechanism and breaking the Valsalva-Stuttering Cycle. We shall call this approach **Valsalva Control**. Unlike previous therapies, which may have had an indirect effect on various steps in the Cycle, Valsalva Control focuses directly on the Valsalva mechanism itself and attacks *all six steps* of the Valsalva-Stuttering Cycle.

Although Valsalva Control is experimental, I believe it is worthy of serious consideration. After decades of failed therapies, this was the approach that finally gave me a "handle" to my own stuttering, enabling me to achieve a dramatic and lasting improvement in fluency. But my good results are not the only justification for this approach. I realize that one person's success is no proof that the same method will help others. For this reason, I have gone far beyond my own personal experience to provide a broad scientific basis for the ideas expressed. Consequently, Valsalva Control is built on a comprehensive theoretical foundation that may reasonably apply to *all* developmental stutterers who exhibit the most common forms of stuttering behavior (*i.e.,* forceful closures and difficulty in phonation).

I am not saying that Valsalva Control is the *only* approach that might be helpful in controlling stuttering, or that it is necessarily the best approach for everybody. If you are having success with a particular technique, stick with it. If you like a particular method but feel it's not helping enough, perhaps Valsalva Control can supply what's missing.

The suggestions in this book are not cast in stone. They can be modified or combined with other methods to suit your individual needs. The extent to which they will prove helpful is a question only you can answer.

Who Might Benefit

Valsalva Control is intended for confirmed stutterers who have been struggling for some time with the ordinary, developmental type of stuttering, characterized by forceful closures and difficulty in phonation. As we know, developmental stuttering usually starts between ages 2 and 8 (although it can begin much later in some cases) and covers the vast majority of people who stutter.

However, Valsalva Control may not be appropriate for people with other types of stuttering, or with serious neurological deficits. Nor would it apply to vocal problems such as spasmodic dysphonia (a neurological condition affecting the vocal cords). Such conditions may require treatment of a totally different nature. Therefore, if you are not certain that your condition is ordinary developmental stuttering, see a speech pathologist or medical specialist (e.g., a neurologist or laryngologist) for a proper diagnosis.

Furthermore, Valsalva Control is not intended for young children who are just beginning to stutter. As we have seen, the factors that cause a child's original disfluency may be different from those that perpetuate stuttering in older children and adults. Today there are "stuttering intervention" programs designed to nip early stuttering in the bud, before it becomes entrenched. Our approach, on the other hand, is aimed at older children, teenagers, and adults, whose stuttering has become a deeply rooted behavior.

Objectives of Valsalva Control

The purpose of Valsalva Control is to unlock the stutterer's inherent fluency by reducing the Valsalva mechanism's interference with speech. Unlike the "fluency training" types of therapies, we do not view stuttering as being a problem with your speech mechanism. Therefore, we will not insist that you trade your natural speaking ability for an artificial-sounding technique that allegedly keeps you from stuttering. Although our suggested exercises may use some fluency enhancing methods (such as airflow and continuous phonation), the ultimate focus will be on *controlling the Valsalva mechanism*, thereby allowing you to speak in a free and natural way.

This will be a gradual process, requiring a complete reprogramming of your reaction to speaking situations, on both physical and psychological levels. Valsalva Control offers no quick "cure," no magic trick that guarantees perfect fluency forever. Rather, it is a rational approach to controlling stuttering based on an understanding of the Valsalva Hypothesis, as explained in the earlier parts of this book. It involves attitude changes (to be discussed in Chapters 24 and 28), exercises in Valsalva control (Chapter 25) and phonation (Chapter 26), as well as recommended speaking techniques (Chapter 27). Like any new skill, it will demand continual practice on a daily basis.

The Fluency Cycle

Valsalva Control is organized around six basic rules, each designed to counteract specific steps of the Valsalva-Stuttering Cycle. Together, these rules form their own self-reinforcing circle, which we shall call the **Fluency Cycle**. They are:

Rule 1. Develop a positive attitude toward speech.

The first step in the Valsalva-Stuttering Cycle is the expectation, either conscious or unconscious, that speaking will be difficult. The various factors that may contribute to such an expectation have been discussed in Chapters 11, 12, and 13. This anticipation of difficulty sets off a chain of psychological, neurological, and physical reactions that lead to stuttering.

Therefore, you need to replace these negative attitudes with a positive anticipation of speech. Instead of preparing for the worst, *look forward to speaking as an easy and pleasant experience*. Rather than worrying about stuttering, *accept the fact that you stutter sometimes and don't try to hide it*. These attitude changes are fundamental to a reversal of the Valsalva-Stuttering Cycle. They will not come easily, but must evolve over time, as you build up your confidence by repeated use of the Fluency Cycle.

Rule 2. Resist the urge to "try hard" in speaking.

In response to the anticipation of difficulty, stutterers may feel that physical effort is needed to force out the words. As a part of your attitude change, you must *root out any urge to "try hard" in speaking*. You must recognize that fluent speech needs very little effort and that "trying hard" only interferes with fluency.

Another aspect of this problem, discussed in previous chapters, is the possibility that stutterers treat words as if they were "things" that can be physically "forced out" by means of a Valsalva maneuver. In order to avoid this tendency, learn to *treat words as phonation and a sequence of movements, rather than as "things" to be forced out*. An exercise called **Adronian speech** will be described in Chapter 26 to help you in this task.

Rule 3. Relax the Valsalva mechanism — don't force!

As discussed in Chapter 7, the stutterer's urge

to force out the words is translated by the brain into neuromotor tuning signals that put the Valsalva mechanism into a heightened state of excitability. When this happens, the entire mechanism is prepared to perform a Valsalva maneuver the instant a triggering stimulus is received. The larynx is ready for effort closure, rather than phonation, while the chest, abdominal, and rectal muscles are poised to contract in unison.

A key objective of Valsalva Control is to prevent Valsalva tuning from occurring. One strategy will be to "tune down" the Valsalva mechanism by *relaxing the muscles that comprise it.* I have found that is best accomplished by focusing on a few specific muscles farthest removed from the movements of speech — namely the abdominal and rectal muscles. Relaxing them tends to relax the entire Valsalva mechanism as well. One of our suggestions will be to *relax your abdomen and rectal muscles, and feel the relaxation spread through your body, all the way to your larynx.*

Breathing methods can also relax the Valsalva mechanism. The technique we shall suggest is to *take a full breath, using the diaphragm, and then relax the abdomen as you exhale.*

As we saw in Chapter 8, a Valsalva maneuver may be triggered by the increases in air pressure caused by routine closures of the mouth or larynx during speech. You can reduce this risk if you *breathe and speak in ways that avoid abrupt increases in air pressure.* Several existing techniques may help in this regard, such as passive airflow, easy onset when starting phonation, and light contacts of the lips and tongue while articulating. These will be incorporated into our suggestions for speaking, to be found in Chapter 27. As we shall also point out, speech tends to be more manageable and less stressful when you *speak in short phrases* and plan ahead for regular pauses in which to breathe.

Rule 4. Focus on phonation and vowels.

Fluency can be enhanced by methods that focus your attention on phonation or that emphasize the vowel sounds of speech. There may be two reasons behind this beneficial effect:
• First, concentrating on voice may cause the brain to *"tune up" the larynx for phonation rather than effort closure.* This would help to relax the Valsalva mechanism and reduce the likelihood of Valsalva tuning.
• Second, this approach may help to avoid the delays in phonation that are a major component of stuttering behavior. For these reasons, it is important, while speaking, to *pay attention to the music and resonance of your voice.* Phonation can be further emphasized if you *intentionally stretch or prolong words or syllables* — a technique that may help when you feel you are going to block.

In Chapter 26, we shall suggest exercises and techniques aimed at improving phonation and keeping the vocal cords ready at all times. One of our principal exercises, called Adronian speech, will combine phonation with several other elements of Valsalva Control.

Rule 5. Speak slowly and deliberately, without avoidance.

Slow and deliberate speech has been one of the most common and effective ways of improving fluency, as we discussed in Chapter 17. Often stutterers try to speak too fast, as if racing to get the words out before stuttering catches up with them. This increases the difficulty of speech, as well as the tendency to use excessive force and to block.

Slowed speech reduces this pressure. It is calming and relaxing. It allows you to set your own pace. Among other benefits, it simplifies the mechanics of speech by stretching words out into a more easily handled sequence of movements. This may reduce the feeling of difficulty and the urge to force out the words as if they were "things." In addition, the slowing of speech increases the emphasis on vowel sounds, thereby enhancing phonation.

This rule also seeks to eliminate the many varieties of avoidance behavior (described in Chapter 10) with which stutterers attempt to hide, postpone, or avoid their blocks. As long as you hide behind avoidance tactics, it will be difficult to recognize and deal with the underlying tendency to block. In Chapter 25, we shall suggest an exercise, called **Voluntary Valsalva**, to help you confront the underlying blocks directly, rather than avoiding them.

Another form of avoidance is the tendency of many stutterers to look away from their listeners while stuttering. This is unfortunate, because it destroys personal communication and leaves the stutterer alone in his struggle. Therefore, a simple but effective rule is to *keep eye contact with the listener, even if you are blocking.* Eye contact may help to reduce the blocks by reminding you of the real purpose of speech — communication.

Rule 6. View your speech objectively.

The final step in the Fluency Cycle is to eliminate the negative reactions you may have to your stuttering. This is aimed at counteracting Step 6 of the Valsalva-Stuttering Cycle, in which the speaker views stuttering as confirming his original belief that speech would be difficult. Stutterers may also get the false impression that their excessive effort ultimately succeeded in forcing the words out.

We shall deal with these negative reactions in Chapter 28, encouraging you to view your speech objectively, to learn from your speaking experiences, both fluent and disfluent, and to maintain your self-esteem, regardless of fluency.

The Road to Improvement

Just as the Valsalva-Stuttering Cycle is a self-perpetuating, self-reinforcing circle, the Fluency Cycle is also a circle. But rather than being vicious, it is revitalizing. Each step in the Fluency Cycle has a positive effect that naturally leads into the next one.

For example, when you look forward to speaking as an easy and pleasant experience (Rule 1), you will have less of an urge to "try hard" to force out the words as if they were "things." When you don't feel the urge to force out the words, your brain will be less likely to "tune up" your Valsalva mechanism. Without Valsalva tuning, your vocal cords will be freer to phonate, and there will be less chance that increases in air pressure during speech will trigger a Valsalva maneuver that blocks speech. With less tendency to block, you will have less temptation to use avoidance behaviors. With less blocking and stuttering, your reaction to your speech is bound to be more positive. Finally, a successful speaking experience will show that speech is not so difficult after all, thereby completing the circle by strengthening your positive attitude in Rule 1.

As you go around the Fluency Cycle the first few times, not much will seem to change. Your desire to view speech positively may seem contrary to your actual experiences. Your attempts to control the Valsalva mechanism may seem hopeless in the face of its long-established power. As you continue to block, you may be tempted to abandon this approach as just another failure. But don't be discouraged.

Instead of looking for immediate results, you should begin by treating the Fluency Cycle as a *tool for learning.* Your use of the Fluency Cycle will go through several phases:

• First, as you concentrate on each step in the Fluency Cycle, *become aware of the opposite things that you think and do.* Don't just take your old attitudes and behaviors for granted. Take a good look at how they interfere with your speech by perpetuating the Valsalva-Stuttering Cycle.

• Then, begin the process of changing those attitudes and behaviors, replacing them with ones that promote fluency. This must be done gradually, paying attention to all six points in the Cycle. It will require continuous dedication, repeated practice, and the use of exercises such as those suggested in the following chapters. As the changes slowly take hold, notice how they tend to make speech easier and more fluent.

• When stuttering returns — as it inevitably will from time to time — don't consider this a failure. Instead, *learn* from the experience. Go back and examine what you were thinking and doing when you blocked. See what aspects of the Valsalva-Stuttering Cycle were involved and understand how they contributed to the relapse. Whatever you do, *never give in to the temptation to try harder!* Increasing the amount of effort will throw your speech right back into the jaws of the Valsalva mechanism, killing any chance of progress.

• Finally, you must learn to consolidate your control over the Valsalva mechanism and extend it to more and more speaking situations.

In the next chapter, we shall begin our quest for change by exploring ways to develop a Valsalva-free attitude toward speech.

THE FLUENCY CYCLE

1. Develop a positive attitude toward speech.
Look forward to speaking as an easy and pleasant experience. Accept the fact that you stutter sometimes, and don't try to hide it.

6. View your speech objectively, without shame or blame.
Learn from your speaking experiences, both fluent and disfluent. Don't be fooled into thinking that force or avoidance helped to get the words out. Speak as much as possible. Maintain your self-esteem.

2. Resist the urge to "try hard."
Remember that fluent speech requires very little physical effort. Effort never helps to get the words out, and only serves to block them. Learn to treat words as phonation and a sequence of movements.

5. Speak slowly and deliberately, without avoidance.
Don't try to rush the words out. Don't hide behind avoidance tactics. Go ahead and say what you want, without substitutions or backtracking. Keep eye contact with the listener, even if you are blocking.

3. Relax the Valsalva mechanism — don't force!
Relax your abdomen and rectal muscles, and feel the relaxation spread through your body, all the way to your larynx. Take a full breath, using your diaphragm, and relax your abdomen as you exhale. Keep an open larynx. Don't hold your breath. Speak each phrase at the same time as you relax your abdomen. Speak in short phrases. Use passive airflow, light contacts, and easy onset to avoid building up air pressure. Again: **don't force!**

4. Focus on phonation and vowels.
Pay attention to the music and resonance of your voice. Keep a relaxed, open larynx, with vocal cords ready to phonate. Concentrate on phonation, using variations in pitch and inflection. Intentionally stretch or prolong syllables when necessary.

CHAPTER 24.

Adopting a Valsalva-Free Attitude

FLUENCY TECHNIQUES will have little value as long as we harbor attitudes that make Valsalva tuning almost inevitable. Beliefs about the difficulty of speech and the need to "try hard" are what set the Valsalva-Stuttering Cycle in motion. Therefore, an essential part of Valsalva Control is to challenge all the assumptions about speech and stuttering that we have accumulated through the years.

Speech itself is not difficult. What is difficult is changing our attitudes and behaviors that *make* speech difficult.

If you are like me, some of these attitudes date back to childhood, when stuttering first began. They are so long-standing that we rarely bother to question them. We unconsciously accept them as immutable facts of life, like gravity. However, they are the ground in which the Valsalva-Stuttering Cycle is rooted. We must now replace them with attitudes that are "Valsalva-free."

Identify Your Negative Attitudes

The first step in the Valsalva-Stuttering Cycle is the expectation that speaking will be difficult, or that a particular word or sound will be hard to say. There is probably no stutterer in the world who doesn't have such a negative anticipation, at least on an unconscious level.

Any number of factors may contribute to the expectation of difficulty, depending on the individual and the speaking situation. Some of these have been discussed in previous chapters. They may include:
• The memory of past experiences in which speaking was difficult;
• Excessive concern about the importance of good speech;
• Fear of stuttering;
• Fear of specific speaking situations;
• Uncertainty, emotional conflict, or ambivalence about talking;
• A feeling of impaired speaking ability due to fatigue, illness, inexperience, or other factors; and
• One's self-image as a stutterer.

Before these attitudes can be changed, we must be able to identify them and recognize the pernicious ways in which they interfere with our preparation for speech. The next time you feel anxious about a speaking situation, stop for a moment and notice what you are thinking.

Are you thinking about how hard it will be to get the words out? Are you especially worried about saying certain words or sounds? Are you expecting to be judged according to your fluency or stuttering — as if speech were a test of your worthiness as a person? Are you viewing the prospect of speaking as a painful struggle, an up hill battle?

For confirmed stutterers, thoughts like these may become so entrenched that they are accepted as self-evident truths. Their validity seems to be reaffirmed, time and again, by the whole agonizing experience of stuttering. However, they should not be taken at face value. As we have seen, the expectation of difficulty may become a self-fulfilling prophesy by setting in motion the Valsalva-Stuttering Cycle. Such thoughts are *not* true reflections of how speech has to be. On the contrary, they are part of the problem.

Much has been written about the "self-talk" that constantly goes on in our minds, and how these internal dialogues affect the way we feel and behave. The same is true in stuttering. Therefore, in order to change our attitudes we must:
- Be aware of the negative things we are telling ourselves;
- Recognize their false and self-defeating nature; and
- Replace them with positive statements that will help us relax our Valsalva mechanism and deal more effectively with speaking situations.[1]

If your sense of difficulty is aggravated by emotional conflicts or other fears or ambivalence about speaking, you may have to dig deep into your feelings and memories to figure out what's bothering you. This may require, in appropriate cases, the help of a psychotherapist to sort things out. However, psychotherapy should not be seen as a cure for stuttering itself. As we have repeatedly pointed out, emotional conflict is only one of many factors that may influence stuttering.

Look Forward to Speaking

The first rule of the Fluency Cycle is to *develop a positive attitude toward speech*. Of course, your deep-seated negative attitudes won't be changed overnight. They must be continually challenged, again and again, as part of a systematic attack on the entire Valsalva-Stuttering Cycle. The goal is to create an attitude in which you *look forward to speaking as an easy and pleasant experience*.

You might start the process by searching your memory for speaking experiences that were enjoyable — *even if you weren't fluent*. Recall the fun you had conversing with your family, friends, or other people. Think of the satisfaction you felt when you spoke your mind, when you shared your ideas and feelings.

Good memories may, at first, seem few and far between. However, they are bound to increase if you stop judging your speaking experiences according to fluency and concentrate instead on their enjoyable aspects. Likewise, when you speak, focus on the pleasure you can have, whether or not you stutter.

Whenever you can, practice speaking just for the fun of it. You might read poetry or dramatic speeches aloud to yourself or into a tape recorder. Put expression and feeling into your readings. Let yourself be a "ham."[2] Take pleasure in the music and resonance of your voice. Experiment with various kinds of intonation and emphasis. Sense the way your mouth caresses the words as they are formed.

Look for opportunities to speak in a relaxed, supportive environment. An ideal place may be a self-help support group, such as the NSA. If there is one in your area, go to the meetings. Participate in the discussions. Get up and give extemporaneous speeches to the group.

Feel good about yourself for speaking, regardless of your fluency. Remember, *speech is not a test of your worthiness*. It's simply a method of communication, which you are entitled to use as much as anyone else. So don't take it so seriously. Be playful about it and lighten up. No law says that you must constantly beat up on yourself for stuttering.

Accept the Fact that You Stutter

If you are to control your stuttering, you must first be willing to accept its existence and look at it objectively. Some stutterers feel that stuttering is too shameful and degrading to own up to. They go to desperate lengths to pretend that it's not really happening. I myself have tried this in the past. Whenever I started to block, my mind went into what's been called "the stutterer's fog." I momentarily "switched channels," so to speak, to avoid dealing with reality. This simply made my listener feel more uncomfortable than ever and destroyed any chance of honest communication.

The more I tried to deny my stuttering, the more I abdicated control of the situation. By closing my eyes to what was actually going on, I never learned a damn thing. I let myself get sucked into a blind struggle to "stop stuttering," in which I kept making the same mistakes over and over again. I let myself become a helpless victim of the Valsalva-Stuttering Cycle.

When viewed objectively, there is nothing

shameful about stuttering. It is not a sign that we are crazy, defective, or unworthy. According to the Valsalva Hypothesis, stuttering may result from a confusion between two otherwise normal bodily functions — the voice and the Valsalva mechanism. This now provides a possible explanation for stuttering that you can discuss with other people without any cause for embarrassment.

Accepting your stuttering doesn't mean giving up your desire to be fluent. On the contrary, it makes fluency more attainable. When you are less fearful of stuttering, you reduce, to some degree, your anticipation of difficulty (which is Step 1 in the Valsalva-Stuttering Cycle). Acceptance allows you to observe and understand your stuttering behavior in a constructive way. Furthermore, being honest with yourself about this important aspect of your life can be the foundation of genuine self-esteem and personal power.

Some years ago, I composed a statement called "A Stutterer's Declaration," for use at our local chapter meetings. It is reproduced in the box below. It summarizes the kind of constructive attitude that can facilitate change.

A Stutterer's Declaration

My name is _____*.*

I am a person who stutters.

I can live with that, and so can you.

I'm not afraid to stutter,

And I'm not afraid to change,

As every day I learn more and more control.

Visualize Your Speaking Role

Visualization can be a powerful tool for improving one's attitude toward speech. In this technique, you create a detailed mental image of yourself in various speaking situations.[3] The object of this exercise is to imagine all of the enjoyable and rewarding aspects of talking with other people — without any regard to stuttering. You should *not* try to picture yourself being fluent, at least in the beginning, because this may be an unrealistic goal that only increases your anxiety.

Instead, your mental picture should focus on the underlying *role* that you are playing, while giving yourself permission to stutter all you want. For example, if you are going to perform a role on stage, you should imagine yourself as actually *being* the character — while at the same time pretending that the character is *supposed* to be someone who stutters. If you are giving a sales promotion, imagine that you are a very effective salesperson — who just happens to stutter.

I have found this approach to be quite valuable during my legal career. When I first prepared to represent clients in court, I managed to subdue my fear of stuttering by concentrating on my role as a lawyer. I said to myself: "I am an *advocate*. I may be a stammering advocate, but, first and foremost, *I am an advocate!*" My zest for being a trial lawyer ultimately swept aside any concern about stuttering, allowing me to perform effectively in many trials and other challenging situations.[4]

Resist the Urge To "Try Hard"

Perhaps the greatest misconception to plague stutterers is the notion that physical effort will help them to speak fluently. I have been painfully aware of this tendency in myself. When I anticipated difficulty, I would hit the "panic button." I would be gripped by the overwhelming urge to force out the words. Somehow, this felt like the only way to salvation. The very notion of *not* using effort seemed too frightening to contemplate.

Using effort may seem like the "good" and conscientious thing to do. It may relieve our feelings of guilt by showing people how *hard* we're trying to get the words out. However, in reality this attitude is self-defeating. It only increases our tendency to activate the Valsalva mechanism, which leads to the blockage of speech.

As we have seen, fluent speech requires very little effort. No matter how difficult the speaking situation seems, effort *never* helps to get the words out — it only serves to block them in. Therefore, as stated in Rule 2 of the Fluency Cycle, you must *resist the urge to "try hard" in speaking.*

This is one of the most crucial things you can do to control stuttering — and perhaps the most difficult. When the "moment of truth" arrives, the urge to use force may feel overwhelming, the idea of speech without effort may seem impossible. It may take courage not to hit the panic button. Nevertheless, you must "say no" to your old habits of struggle and learn a new response to speaking situations. This will include the relaxation of your Valsalva mechanism.

Treat Words as Phonation and Movement

The way we look at words may have a subtle but profound effect on how we process speech. In previous chapters, we explored the possibility that stutterers tend to view words as if they were "things" — solid objects that could be held in the mouth like jaw-breaker candy, or forced out of the body with the help of a Valsalva maneuver. Indeed, that seems to be the way stutterers actually *treat* words during speech. Therefore, it's reasonable to suppose that stutterers might *think* about words in the same way.

Viewing words as "things" may increase our tendency to activate the Valsalva mechanism. As we recall from Chapter 6, one of the normal uses of a Valsalva maneuver is for bearing down during defecation. We instinctively used the Valsalva maneuver to help us force out bowel movements as little children. When we experienced disfluency, perhaps we felt that our difficulty in getting the words out was a kind of "verbal constipation" — which we then tried to overcome by using the Valsalva mechanism.

The fact you must keep in mind was expressed most memorably by a psychiatrist-speech pathologist to whom I mentioned this idea some years ago. "Then what the stutterer must come to realize," he remarked, "is that *words are not turds!*"

Precisely.

Words should be treated instead as what they are: voiced sounds (phonation) and a sequence of movements (articulation). Imagine speech as a ballet — a coordination of music and dance. Your voice is the music. Against this background, your lips and tongue do a graceful dance of articulation, like ballerinas tiptoeing lightly about.

Other Changes

Many other attitudes — about speech, stuttering, and ourselves — will have to be changed before the Valsalva-Stuttering Cycle is dislodged by the Fluency Cycle.[5] But these psychological changes must go hand in hand with *physical* changes in our behavior before and during speech. Therefore, we shall postpone further discussion of attitudes until Chapter 28, and turn now to exercises aimed at controlling the Valsalva mechanism.

Notes

1. For detailed advice on how to replace negative self-talk with effective self-talk in controlling stuttering, see Webster, W. G., & Poulos, M. G., *Facilitating Fluency: Transfer Strategies for Adult Stuttering Treatment Programs,* 5th ed, Edmonton, AB: Institute for Stuttering Treatment & Research, 1997 (reformatted and reprinted from 1989 work of the same title originally published by Communication Skill Builders, Tucson, AZ).

2. You may wish to try some of the public speaking exercises found in Harrison, J. C., *How To Conquer Your Fears of Speaking Before People,* 5th ed, Anaheim Hills, CA: Nat'l Stuttering Ass'n, 1999.

3. Some persons who stutter have told me that they have benefitted from the relaxation and visualization techniques found in Maltz, M., *Psycho-Cybernetics* (Hollywood, CA: Wilshire Book Co., 1960).

4. As we shall discuss further in Chapter 28, the real obstacle is not fear itself, but the way we have learned to *react* to fear. See Jeffers, S., *Feel the Fear and Do It Anyway,* New York: Fawcett Columbine, 1987.

5. John Harrison, Program Director of the National Stuttering Association, has envisioned stuttering as an interactive system involving a number of different components, which he has called "The Stuttering Hexagon." Its six components are *speech behaviors, emotions, perceptions, beliefs, intentions,* and *genetics.* Except for the genetic factor, which is constant, each of the other elements reinforces all the others, thereby perpetuating the system. Therefore, a change in only one of these components is not likely to last very long unless the other components are changed also. Harrison, J. C., Developing a new paradigm for stuttering, *How To Conquer Your Fears of Speaking Before People,* 5th ed, Anaheim Hills, CA: Nat'l Stuttering Ass'n, 1999.

CHAPTER 25.

Exercises for Valsalva Control

THE EXERCISES IN THIS CHAPTER are to acquaint you with your Valsalva mechanism, to give you a feeling of how it can block your speech, and to teach you how to create and release these blocks at will. We shall then move on to ways of "tuning down" the Valsalva mechanism through relaxation and breathing methods.

Before beginning, it might be helpful to review Chapter 6, which explains the Valsalva mechanism and the Valsalva maneuver in more detail.

The Valsalva Maneuver

We shall start by introducing the normal function of the Valsalva mechanism — the performance of a basic Valsalva maneuver.

Inhale, and then hold your breath. Gradually build up air pressure, as if you are straining to lift a heavy weight. Continue to strain to a moderate degree, without causing yourself to feel uncomfortable. (Don't overdo it, particularly if you have a heart condition, because in extreme cases a person might pass out.) Hold that position for a moment, and become aware of the muscles and parts of your body that feel tense or constricted.

Notice that your larynx is tightly closed. It is blocking your upper airway to keep air from getting out. This is a normal function of the larynx called **effort closure**. At the same time, muscles around your mid-section and abdomen are extremely tense and contracted. These muscles are squeezing to build up air pressure in the lungs. The harder they squeeze, the tighter your larynx blocks the upper airway to keep the air from escaping. This simultaneous blockage of the upper airway and contraction of the chest and abdominal muscles is what we know as a Valsalva maneuver.

If you pay careful attention, you may notice that your rectal muscles are also tense. They are squeezing the rectum to prevent the pressure from accidentally causing an evacuation of the bowels.

All of these parts of the body — the larynx, certain chest muscles, abdominal muscles, and rectal muscles — are part of the Valsalva mechanism. They are neurologically coordinated to contract at the same time to do a Valsalva maneuver. In other words, if you tighten one part of the Valsalva mechanism, the other parts will have a natural tendency to tighten also.

Notice how the more you strain, the more tightly your throat closes. As discussed in Chapter 6, the increase in air pressure automatically stimulates the Valsalva mechanism to block the upper airway with greater force in order to hold the air in.

Stopping the Maneuver. Now see what happens when you *stop* doing the Valsalva maneuver. First, your abdominal and chest muscles *relax*. Once they stop squeezing and the air pressure goes down, the larynx automatically relaxes and allows the air to flow freely.

Blocking with the Mouth. The larynx is not the only structure that may be used by the Valsalva mechanism to block the airway. As we have previously shown, the Valsalva mechanism can also use the *mouth* (either the lips or tongue) to block the airway. We shall now do some more Valsalva exercises to demonstrate.

Put your lips together as if forming the letter *p*. Now do the strongest block you can. Notice how your abdominal and chest muscles have tightened to build up air pressure. Feel how your lips press together with ever greater force the more you strain. You are doing a Valsalva maneuver. Now relax your abdominal muscles. Notice how, when the air pressure decreases, your lips automatically relax also. The block disappears.

Repeat the same exercise while putting your lips and tongue in different positions. For example, start by touching the tip of your tongue to gum ridge behind your upper teeth, as if forming a *t* sound. Now when you do a Valsalva maneuver, feel how the muscles of the tongue tighten up to block the airway. Relax your abdomen and see how the tongue also relaxes.

Next, begin by raising the back of your tongue to the roof of your mouth, as if forming a *k* sound. Now the Valsalva maneuver causes that portion of the tongue to press tightly. Again relax your abdomen and see how this relaxes your tongue.

These exercises demonstrate a fundamental principle: *You can't do a forceful block (or a Valsalva maneuver) while relaxing your abdomen.*

Voluntary Valsalva

In our next exercise, you will intentionally duplicate the Valsalva blocks during speech. This will, in effect, be a kind of voluntary stuttering, which we call **Voluntary Valsalva**. One objective is to gain control of the involuntary spasms by learning how to create them and release them on purpose.

Instead of repeating the beginning sound of a word, as in voluntary controlled repetition ("VCR"), you will *silently* block on the word by doing a Valsalva maneuver. After blocking and building up air pressure, you will then release the block by *relaxing your abdomen*. This will reduce the air pressure, which will tend to relax the mouth or larynx and let speech flow more freely.

Peter Piper. Let's try this out with the old tongue-twister, "Peter Piper." Intentionally block on every *p* sound, doing a Valsalva maneuver at each asterisk (*). Press the lips together, build up air pressure, and then relax your abdomen to release the block. When the air finally comes out, it should *not* be in an explosive burst, but rather in a gentle flow.

P*eter P*iper p*icked a p*eck of p*ickled p*eppers.
A p*eck of p*ickled p*eppers P*eter P*iper p*icked.
If P*eter P*iper p*icked a p*eck of p*ickled p*eppers.
Where's the p*eck of p*ickled p*eppers P*eter P*iper p*icked?

Other Sounds. Now try Voluntary Valsalva while reading other material, such as this book or a newspaper. Try blocking on every *p* you come to. Then try other plosives, such as every *b*, hard *c*, *d*, hard *g*, *k*, *p*, and *t*.

Next, try blocking on initial *vowel* sounds, such as the *a* in "apple." For these sounds, it is the larynx that squeezes shut. Read aloud some more, this time blocking on every word that starts with a vowel — closing the larynx tightly and then relaxing your abdomen to release the sound.

The plosives and initial vowels are the best sounds on which to practice Voluntary Valsalva, because the airway is completely closed and the block is silent. Other consonants are not as good for this purpose, because the air is only partially blocked, resulting in a prolonged sound. These include the fricatives (*f, h, j, s, sh, th, v,* and *z*), the liquids (*l* and *r*), and the semi-vowels (*w* and *y*).

However, you can practice blocking on these sounds also, if you wish. Even though the air pressure does not build up as much as in the case of plosives, you will find that the blocks can still be released by relaxing your abdomen.

Going Public. After you have mastered Voluntary Valsalva in private, try it while speaking to other people. Start with a friend or relative, or members of your stuttering support group, if you belong to one. These people should be told the object of the exercise and should encourage you to block frequently when you forget to do it. They can also give feedback on how well you are relaxing the blocks, to make sure that the air is being released gently, with reduced pressure, and not explosively.

The next phase of practice will be to take Voluntary Valsalva into the real world. Chances

Chapter 25 / Exercises for Valsalva Control

are you will feel somewhat embarrassed and reluctant to do this. So we suggest you begin with situations in which you feel relatively anonymous — for example, ordering food in a restaurant where you don't know anyone, speaking to sales clerks in stores you don't ordinarily frequent, or calling for routine information on the telephone.

Benefits. Although I am not a fan of voluntary stuttering in its VCR form, I believe that Voluntary Valsalva can serve some useful purposes. It may, for example:

• Put you more in control of your tendency to block, by demonstrating what a block is and how to get out of it;

• Desensitize you somewhat from the fear of stuttering;

• Cut through the use of avoidance behaviors; and

• Provide valuable practice in releasing Valsalva maneuvers during speech by relaxing the abdomen.

Valsalva Relaxation

Now that you are familiar with Valsalva maneuvers and how to release them, we shall turn to exercises aimed at relaxing the Valsalva mechanism *before* speech begins. The purpose is to neurologically "tune down" the Valsalva mechanism, making it less excitable and less likely to interfere with phonation or cause blocks.

Targets for Relaxation. I have found that it's easier to keep the Valsalva mechanism relaxed if you focus on *a single point* within it. Because the Valsalva muscles are neurologically coordinated, tensing or relaxing even *one* of them will affect the entire Valsalva mechanism. The trick, however, is to find a Valsalva muscle that is easily distinguishable from other muscles that are normally active during speech.

For this reason, the larynx is probably *not* a good place to begin. It contains more than a dozen little muscles — some for phonation, some for effort closure, and some for both. Targeting an appropriate Valsalva muscle in the larynx would be difficult due to this complexity.

Relaxing the abdomen is crucial, especially while exhaling when you start to speak. However, there are times when some muscles in the abdomen are actively involved in breathing.

As bizarre as it may seem, a good muscle to relax is probably found in the *rectum*. Specifically, we are referring to the **puborectalis muscle**, which is located inside your body, an inch or two above the anus. It forms a sling around the rectum, the passageway between the intestines and the anus. During a Valsalva maneuver, it pinches the rectum shut to prevent accidental evacuation of the bowels. (It would not contract, however, if you *intended* to move your bowels.) The rectal muscle may be an ideal target for relaxation, because it is far removed from any activity involving speech or breathing.

The effect of the rectal muscle on the Valsalva mechanism is something you can experience yourself. Begin by voluntarily tightening your rectum, As you do, your larynx will probably have a tendency to close automatically. Now relax your rectum. Feel how the larynx relaxes into an open position.

I confirmed this phenomenon for myself during the nasopharyngoscopic study described in Chapter 7. On the video monitor, I could actually *see* my larynx close and then open as I tightened and relaxed my rectum.

Relaxation procedure. The following suggestion will borrow one of the techniques from Jacobson's progressive relaxation methods — namely, the practice of tensing the muscle in question before relaxing it.

Gradually *contract* your rectal muscle, to familiarize yourself with the feeling of increased tension. Focus all your attention on that muscle.

Next, reverse the process by gradually *relaxing* the muscle. Continue to relax it slowly, familiarizing yourself with what it feels like to reduce the tension. Return the muscle to the same level of tension as when you started, and then keep going *past* that point, relaxing it more and more. Concentrate on the feeling of greater and greater relaxation in the rectum. The entire rectal area, including the anus, should feel relaxed and open.

Now feel the relaxation spread upward through your abdomen, through your chest, and all the way to your larynx. The larynx should feel relaxed and open, with air flowing freely through it. Once you get a sense of which laryngeal muscles are relaxing, you may concentrate on relaxing them directly.

Feel how the relaxation continues to spread upward, from your throat to your jaw, your tongue, and your lips. Your mouth will feel loose, relaxed, and open. Savor for a while the feeling of relaxed openness, from your mouth and larynx to your rectum.

Maintaining Valsalva Relaxation

Once you have experienced Valsalva relaxation, hold onto the feeling as long as you can. Through the day, concentrate on the relaxation of your rectal muscle and the openness of your larynx. This should not interfere with any of your normal activities. The Valsalva mechanism can stay relaxed, even when you're talking or doing other things.

Purposely refrain from doing Valsalva maneuvers, even in those activities in which they normally occur. If you're like almost every one, you will have an instinctive tendency to close your larynx and tense your chest and abdomen when exerting effort (such as lifting, pushing, pulling, etc.) or trying to move your bowels. However, you don't really *need* the help of a Valsalva maneuver to do these things. You can override this tendency if you intentionally *keep your larynx open.*

Consciously avoiding Valsalva maneuvers is an exercise that may decrease your feeling of dependence on the Valsalva mechanism, while at the same time increasing your ability to control it voluntarily. This is just another part of the overall campaign to "tune down" your Valsalva mechanism so it will be less likely to interfere with speech.

Abdominal Breathing

Many stutterers develop irregular breathing habits, such as gasping, holding or forcing their breath, or beginning speech with insufficient air in the lungs. Often it appears that breathing has been taken hostage by the Valsalva mechanism or the stutterer's avoidance behaviors.

We shall now suggest a way of breathing that will not only supply the airflow needed for speech, but will also help to relax the Valsalva mechanism. This method should be conscientiously practiced every day until it becomes second nature.

First, you will relax your Valsalva mechanism, using the exercise previously described. Throughout your breathing, you will keep your rectum as relaxed as possible. Give yourself room to breathe by throwing back your shoulders and sticking out your chest, rather than slouching.

Next, you will take a "full breath" — deeper than you probably are used to, but not so deep as to be uncomfortable. You will *inhale by using your diaphragm* rather than your chest muscles. This is called **diaphragmatic** or **abdominal breathing,** as distinguished from chest breathing.

As we explained in Chapter 4, the diaphragm is a dome-shaped muscle between the lungs and the intestines. When it is relaxed, the center of it protrudes up into the chest cavity. When you contract the diaphragm, it tightens up, drawing the center downwards. This enlarges the chest cavity, causing the lungs to expand and draw in air. At the same time, it compresses the abdominal cavity, causing the intestines to protrude outward.

When you relax the diaphragm, the reverse occurs. The muscle returns to its dome-like shape. The center goes back up, making the chest cavity smaller and the abdominal cavity larger. The lungs contract like rubber balloons, releasing a flow of air through the larynx. Meanwhile, the intestines go back into their usual space.

It's easy tell if you're breathing diaphragmatically. Simply observe your abdomen. When you inhale, the displaced intestines will cause the abdomen to protrude outward. When you exhale, the abdomen will go back in. You can monitor this while breathing by placing one hand on the front of your abdomen, right below the beltline. Another way to practice is to lie on your back with a book placed on your abdomen. As you breathe, you will watch the book go up and down.

After inhaling, *don't hold your breath*. Allow your larynx to remain open. You will *exhale by gradually relaxing your abdomen*. As you do so, the diaphragm will also relax, allowing the lungs to contract of their own accord. Relaxing the abdomen will also help to relax the entire Valsalva mechanism.

Do not force the air in any way. It should be completely "passive," flowing gently through your open larynx without any effort on your part. This type of breathing allows the Valsalva mechanism to stay relaxed and avoids any abrupt increases in air pressure that might trigger a Valsalva maneuver.

During actual speech, the chest or abdominal muscles will tend to contract slightly, in order to maintain sufficient airflow to keep the vocal cords vibrating properly (as discussed in Chapter 4). Therefore, technically speaking, your airflow will probably not be *totally* passive. For present purposes, however, you need not worry about this detail. Simply concentrate on keeping your exhalation as relaxed and passive as possible at all times.

We have now combined relaxation of the Valsalva muscles with relaxed abdominal breathing. Next we shall add a third element — phonation — to be discussed in the following chapter.

CHAPTER 26.

Phonation Exercises

BUILDING UPON the Valsalva relaxation and breathing methods described in the previous chapter, we shall now introduce exercises that emphasize the importance of phonation. Their underlying purposes will be:

• To relax the Valsalva mechanism by neurologically "tuning" the larynx for phonation instead of effort closure;

• To increase the vocal cords' readiness to make the voiced sounds of speech; and

• To change the way we process speech, by compelling us to treat words not as "things" to be forced out, but as phonation and a sequence of articulatory movements.

Vocalization Exercises

In every exercise that follows, the first step will be to establish Valsalva relaxation and abdominal breathing, using the methods previously described. Maintain a relaxed rectum and open larynx at all times, and relax your abdomen as you exhale. Feel the gentle flow of air through your larynx. Do this for a few minutes until you are fully relaxed.

Phonation. After you have begun exhaling, slowly bring your vocal cords together across the outward flow of air. Don't hold your breath or interrupt the airflow at any time. As the vocal cords close, the airflow will make them vibrate (phonate), producing a gentle "aaah" sound. Let the sound continue, without forcing your breath, until the air runs out. The sound would look like this written out (with the dots indicating the unvoiced airflow before phonation):

". . . . . Aaaaaaaaaaaaaaaa."

Repeat this exercise for several minutes. As you do, here are some things to focus on:

• Concentrate on the feeling of phonation both in your larynx and your body. Touch your Adam's apple and feel the vibration. As your Valsalva mechanism becomes more and more relaxed, sense the vibrations spreading through your chest and abdomen. You should feel as if your whole body is resonating, like a well-tuned musical instrument.

• Notice how phonation and Valsalva relaxation go hand in hand. Phonating relaxes the Valsalva mechanism, and relaxing the Valsalva mechanism helps you to phonate more easily.

• Learn to associate phonating with relaxing your abdomen at the same time. Link the two events closely in your mind, so that relaxing the abdomen becomes an inseparable part of phonation. Whenever you need to phonate, the effect will then be to relax the Valsalva mechanism.

Monitoring Phonation. You can monitor — and improve — your phonation by means of **enhanced vocal feedback**. As we discussed in Chapter 18, various devices and techniques can increase your awareness of the vibrations in your vocal cords. For example, when you cover the opening of one ear with your fingertip, your phonation will seem louder due to a phenomenon called the **occlusion effect**. You can also place your fingers on the front of your throat and actually *feel* your larynx vibrate as you phonate.

Therefore, while doing these phonation exercises, try placing the tip of your middle finger over the opening of one ear and your thumb on your larynx, in order to get the maximum effect.

Voice and Articulation

We are now ready to add another element to our exercises — the articulatory movements of the lips and tongue.

Vocalize again, making a sustained "aaah" sound as you relax your abdomen. Without interrupting the stream of phonation in any way, purse your lips, as if to make a *w,* and then release them. It should sound something like this:

".... Aaaaawaaaaaaaaa."

There should be no break in the sound at all. Your phonation should be a steady, uninterrupted tone, which does not stop, regardless of what your mouth is doing. This is known as **continuous phonation.**

After you have mastered this simple step, try pursing your lips together several times in succession, like this:

".... Aaawaaawaaawaaaa."

Now, instead of the *w,* try touching your lips lightly together to make a *b* sound, like this:

".... Aaabaaabaaabaaaa."

Next, try the same exercise with other articulatory movements as you continuously phonate. Move your lips and tongue as you would to make the sounds for *d, g, j, l, m, n, r, v, y,* and *z*. (A detailed description of these movements can be found in Chapter 5.)

To do continuous phonation properly, you should *never* interrupt your phonation, not even during articulation. Therefore, all the sounds you make should be *voiced.* You should *not* be hearing any unvoiced consonants, like *c, f, k, p, q, s, t,* or *x,* which are made with the vocal cords open.

An Introduction to Adronian Speech

We now arrive at what I have found to be an extremely useful exercise in Valsalva Control. It combines Valsalva relaxation, abdominal breathing, and continuous phonation with the articulatory movements used to form actual words. I have called it **Adronian speech**, for reasons that will become clear.

The basic steps to Adronian speech are as follows:

1. Maintain Valsalva relaxation and abdominal breathing at all times.

2. Take a breath before each phrase, keeping your larynx open and relaxing your abdomen as you exhale. Never force or hold your breath.

3. Begin by allowing some air to flow passively through your open larynx.

4. Gently close your vocal cords to make an "aaah" sound.

5. While making a continuous, uninterrupted sound of phonation, move your mouth, lips, and tongue as you would to form words.

6. *Do not* interrupt phonation or open your vocal cords at any time, even when you come to consonants that are normally unvoiced. Go through the *motions* of articulation, while maintaining a constant drone of phonation in the background. (Hence the name "Adronian" — "aaah" plus "drone".) This means that all the *unvoiced* consonants will become *voiced* consonants. Some words will sound unusual, but don't worry about it.

7. Within each phrase, link all the words together with continuous phonation. One sound should slide right into the next, without a break. Don't stop phonating until the end of the phrase.

8. Speak slowly, in short phrases. Begin with only one word per phrase. Once you feel comfortable with that, gradually increase the phrases to two, three, or four words. Take a breath between phrases and begin each phrase with an "aaah" sound.

Benefits of Adronian Speech

Although Adronian speech contains many fluency enhancing elements, it is not intended to be a fluency technique for ordinary speaking. (It sounds too peculiar for that.) Rather, it is an exercise to produce gradual, long-term improvements that will carry over into everyday speech.

Adronian speech combines several principles of Valsalva Control. For example, it begins each phrase with passive airflow to avoid abrupt increases in air pressure that might trigger a Valsalva maneuver. Then it emphasizes phonation, which both relaxes the Valsalva mechanism and readies the vocal cords to make voiced sounds promptly.

Please note that the purpose of starting each phrase with an "aaah" is simply to instill the habit of *thinking* phonation before speaking. We do *not* intend that you actually say the "aaah" as a "starter" in normal speech.

Stutterers often worry so much about blocking on articulation that they forget the importance of airflow and phonation. Adronian separates all three elements and puts them into their proper priority — first airflow, then phonation, and only then articulation. (Of course, this is for exercise purposes only. You wouldn't actually spread them out this way in ordinary speech.)

In addition, Adronian speech is intended to change the way in which you process words into speech. As you shall see, Adronian changes the sound of many words. Therefore, you cannot monitor your speech simply by listening for the sounds you are used to. Adronian forces you to disregard what you hear and to pay more attention to what your mouth and vocal cords are actually *doing*. This may reduce your customary reliance on **auditory feedback**, and thereby improve your fluency for reasons that have been discussed in Chapter 18. In this way, Adronian may help you to break the Valsalva-Stuttering Cycle by teaching you to concentrate on the phonation and movements of speech, rather than treating words as "things" to be forced out.

A Word About Voiced and Unvoiced Consonants

Adronian's most distinctive characteristic is the way it makes some words sound totally different than usual. Because phonation is continuous, *all* of the sounds are voiced, even those that normally wouldn't be.

In English, some consonants are spoken with the vocal cords closed (*b, d, g, j, l, m, n, r, v, w, y,* and *z*), called the "voiced consonants." Other consonants are spoken with the vocal cords open (*c, f, h, k, p, q, s, t,* and *x*), called the "unvoiced consonants." Most of the unvoiced consonants have a corresponding voiced consonant that is formed by the lips or tongue in the same way.

In Adronian, all the consonants are voiced, since the voice never stops until the end of a phrase. As a result, every unvoiced consonant is replaced by its corresponding voiced consonant. Take, for example, the letters *p* and *b*. Both are made by placing your lips together and gently blowing them apart with your breath. When you do this with an unvoiced breath, you get the *p* sound. When you do the same thing while using your voice, it turns into a *b* sound. (The voiced-unvoiced relationship between other consonants are shown in the accompanying table.)

To see how this changes the sound of a word, let's examine the name "Peter." Both the *p* and the *t* are unvoiced consonants, normally spoken with the vocal cords open. However, during the continuous phonation of Adronian speech, the *p* will turn into a *b* and the *t* will turn into a *d*. "Peter" will therefore come out as "Beder."

To demonstrate, let's go back to the nursery rhyme "Peter Piper" and hear how it sounds in Adronian. We have written it with the words linked by hyphens. There should be *no pause* after the "aaa" or between any of the words in the phrase. One word should flow right into the next, without any interruption whatsoever. When you

---

Corresponding Voiced and Unvoiced Consonants

The following is a list of unvoiced consonants and the corresponding voiced consonants which replace them. (No, you *don't* have to memorize this!)

Unvoiced	Voiced
c (as in cat)	g
c (as in cent)	z
ch	j
f	v
h	(no voiced consonant; it is replaced by the vowel sound that follows it)
k	g
p	b
ph	v
q	g
s	z
t	d
th (as in thank)	<u>th</u> (as in then)
x	gz

Chapter 26 / Phonation Exercises

come to a slash (/), stop and take a breath.

... Aaaa-Beder-Biber-bigged/
... aaaa-a-beg-ov-biggled-bebberz./
... Aaaa-a-beg-ov-biggled-bebberz/
... aaaa-Beder-Biber-bigged./
... Aaaa-iv-Beder-Biber-bigged/
... aaaa-a-beg-ov-biggled-bebberz/
... aaaa-where'z-the-beg/
... aaaa-ov-biggled-bebberz/
... aaaa-Beder-Biber-bigged?

Practicing Adronian

The mastering of Adronian speech will take some practice. A good starting point may be the material in Appendix A to this book, called "A Voyage to Adronia." This is a whimsical piece, containing sample dialogues and further information about Adronian, which I prepared for our local NSP chapter. Then continue to use Adronian speech while reading aloud from books, newspapers, or magazines.

Problems with Adronian. I have found that some stutterers have a particularly hard time getting the hang of Adronian speech. The most common problem is that they interrupt phonation between words or when they come to a consonant that is usually unvoiced. Their impulse is to open the vocal cords and say the consonant in the ordinary unvoiced way. To do the exercise correctly, you should forget about how words are *supposed* to sound and simply concentrate on phonating continuously while you move your mouth. To check on how well you're doing, cup a hand behind one ear to hear yourself more clearly, or talk into a tape recorder and listen to the results.

Other problems include the tendency to speak with excessive slowness or prolongation, in a monotone, or with too much effort. This is *not* what is intended by the exercise.

Adronian speech should be relaxed and easy. It is intended to *simplify* speech, not to make it more difficult. It should not detract from your basic mode of Valsalva relaxation and abdominal breathing.

The larynx should simply be allowed to do its thing — to phonate on the outward airflow, without interruption. The mouth should simply go through the motions of mouthing the words, without regard to what the larynx is doing. Your speed, phrasing, intonation, and inflection should be the same as natural speech. You should not use extra effort or stretch everything out in a monotone.

If, after trying for a few days, you still find Adronian speech to be difficult, frustrating, or stressful, then this exercise is probably not for you. If you can't feel comfortable and relaxed with it, it will be counter-productive.

If this is the case, simply practice speaking while using the basic Valsalva relaxation techniques. That is:
• Relax your rectum;
• Breathe abdominally;
• Relax your abdomen as you exhale;
• Coordinate your phonation and speech with the relaxation of your abdomen and outward breath; and
• Continue to relax to the extent that you can

Phonation in Ordinary and Adronian Speech

Ordinary Speech

Sound: Peter Piper picked a peck of pickled peppers.
Voice: v vv   v vv   v   vv v v   vv v vvv   v vv

Adronian Speech

Sound: Aaaa-Beder-Biber-bigged-a-begg-ov-biggled-bebberz.
Voice: vvvvvvvvvvvvvvvvvvvvvvvvvvvvvvvvvvvvvvvvvvvvvvvvvv

feel your phonation vibrating through your body, right down to your abdomen and rectum.

Do as much as you can to practice continuous phonation, to the extent that you feel relaxed and comfortable. You can also practice other techniques that emphasize phonation, such as prolonging the first word or syllable of each phrase.

Continued Practice. Because the effects of Adronian speech are gradual and cumulative, you must continue to practice on a regular basis. Preferably, this should be done for half an hour every morning, in accordance with the daily exercise program to be described in the next chapter.

Practice Adronian during the day whenever you can. Driving alone in a car is a good opportunity for reading road signs, billboards, and even license numbers in Adronian. If you're planning to give a speech or deliver an oral report, rehearse it in Adronian a few times.

Other Adronian exercises might be created to duplicate a variety of speaking situations. Perhaps you can enlist a friend or family member to converse with you in Adronian on occasion. If you know other persons who stutter, perhaps you can plan a meeting, party, or other activity, in which you will speak in Adronian to one another for an extended period of time.

Phasing Back into Normal Speech

You are not expected to go around in public speaking Adronian. As previously stated, Adronian is simply an *exercise* — not a speaking technique for general use. Therefore, after you practice reading aloud in Adronian, phase back into ordinary speech in the following gradual steps:

• As you read in Adronian, gradually soften your vocalization of the unvoiced consonants (*c, f, h, k, p, q, s, t,* and *x*) until they sound more natural. We'll call this step **modified Adronian**. Even while making the unvoiced sounds, continue to *think* vocalization, keeping your vocal cords in constant readiness.

• Next, gradually soften and shorten the "aaah" sound at the beginning of each phrase. Get to the point where you *think* the "aaah" sound without actually saying it out loud. Continue to concentrate on phonation and vowel sounds, linking the words together with your voice. Pay attention to the vibration of your larynx and the fullness and melody of your voice. In addition, you should still maintain Valsalva relaxation and abdominal breathing.

We'll call this step **resonant speech**. It is somewhat similar to **legato speech**, in which the words are joined by continuous phonation. You should concentrate on this mode of speaking for the rest of the day.

In the next chapter, we shall suggest a daily exercise program for maintaining Valsalva Control, as well as specific techniques that may be helpful in ordinary speaking situations.

CHAPTER 27.

Valsalva Control for Everyday Speech

YOUR ABILITY TO CONTROL stuttering during the stress of everyday speech will not come from an intellectual understanding of the problem alone. It requires fundamental changes in your attitudes toward speech and your physical and neurological reactions to speaking situations. This transformation will not happen overnight, nor will it come easily.

In order for them to stick, the changes must become indelibly imprinted in the nerve pathways of your brain and body, just as stuttering was. This can only be accomplished through *actual practice* — through the constant repetition of new behavior patterns until they become second nature.

Consequently, we shall begin this chapter by suggesting an exercise program to provide repeated practice of Valsalva Control methods on a daily basis.

A Daily Exercise Program

At the outset, spend a few hours experimenting with the exercises suggested in Chapters 25 and 26 — especially those involving Valsalva relaxation, abdominal breathing, phonation, and Adronian speech. Practice until you have mastered the basic techniques. Then practice these methods for at least 30 minutes every day to "tune" yourself neurologically for greater fluency. The more regularly you practice, the stronger these nerve pathways will become.

Practice in the morning. The best time to practice is in the morning, after you've washed and dressed, but before you get involved in speaking situations. This may mean setting your alarm clock a half hour earlier, but it's well worth it. I have found, in my own case, that morning practice is essential for progress.

Although the evening may *seem* to be a more convenient time to practice, it simply can't compare with the morning in terms of effectiveness. At night, I found that my mind was too tired to concentrate on speech exercises. They put me to sleep. Even worse, practicing before bed had little or no carry-over effect. I would get all tuned up for fluency, with nowhere to use it. By the time I awoke the next morning, the fluent feeling was gone. As I plunged back into the same old hectic routine, my Valsalva mechanism became tense and I stuttered as usual.

In contrast, morning practice allowed me to "tune" myself for the coming day and to carry my practice into actual speaking situations. Of course, I did not always succeed at maintaining fluency at first, but at least I was in a position to learn from my experiences. Within a few months, I noticed a dramatic improvement in my fluency. Within a year, my life had been transformed. These gains, although gradual, have now remained with me for more than 15 years.

A Suggested Routine

Start every day with the following 30-minute routine, which includes exercises in Valsalva relaxation, abdominal breathing, and Adronian speech. Find a private place with a comfortable chair. Select an appropriate book, magazine, or newspaper for reading. Have a clock or watch in clear view so you can time each part of the practice routine, as follows:

1. Loosening Up (1 minute). Take a minute

to loosen up and relax your neck, shoulders, chest, and mouth. For example, you might:

• Tilt your head forward and back and side to side, to stretch your neck muscles;

• Stretch out your arms and extend them backward;

• Hunch up your shoulders and then relax them;

• Open and close your mouth, stretching the jaw and oral muscles.

2. Valsalva Relaxation (1 minute). Follow the procedure for Valsalva relaxation described in Chapter 25. First, tighten your rectal muscle and then relax it. As you concentrate on relaxing the rectum, feel the relaxation spread through your abdomen and chest, up to your larynx. Your larynx should be open and relaxed.

3. Abdominal Breathing (1 minute). While maintaining Valsalva relaxation, begin abdominal breathing (as explained in Chapter 25). Contract your diaphragm to inhale, relax your abdomen as you exhale, and keep your larynx open. Do not hold or force your breath.

4. Vocalization (2 minutes). While continuing both Valsalva relaxation and abdominal breathing, bring your vocal cords together during each outward breath to make a gentle "aaah" sound. Pay attention to the relaxation of your abdomen as you phonate. As you repeat this vocalization exercise, concentrate on the feelings of phonation in your larynx and your body, as it vibrates all the way down to your abdomen and your rectum.

5. Adronian Speech (15 minutes). On top of the Valsalva relaxation, abdominal breathing, and vocalization, you will now add Adronian speech. Read aloud from a book or article, following the procedures discussed in Chapter 26. Remember to:

• Break up each sentence into short phrases, start each phrase with an "aaah," and take a breath between phrases;

• Continue to phonate through the entire phrase, sliding one sound into the next, without interruption; and

• Move your mouth, lips, and tongue the same as you usually would in saying the words, while vocalizing *everything* — even the consonants that are normally unvoiced.

(If you have trouble doing Adronian, don't worry about it. Simply speak in a relaxed way, emphasizing phonation the best you can. Feel the vibrations resonate through your body. Learn to breathe abdominally and to coordinate your speech with the relaxation of your abdomen as you exhale.)

6. Modified Adronian (5 minutes). Begin to mold Adronian into natural-sounding speech. As mentioned in Chapter 26, the first step will be to decrease gradually your vocalization of the unvoiced consonants until they sound more usual. Nevertheless, you should continue to *think* phonation, even while making the unvoiced sounds.

7. Resonant Speech (5 minutes). For the final 5 minutes, gradually soften and shorten the "aaah" sound at the beginning of each phrase. Reach the point where you *think* the "aaah" sound without actually saying it. (Remember: the purpose is to prepare yourself to phonate, *not* to say "aaah" as a starter.) All of the other elements will continue, including Valsalva relaxation, abdominal breathing, and your emphasis on phonation to link the words together. At this point you should be talking with relaxed, resonant, natural-sounding speech.

Maintenance During the Day

The half-hour morning exercise is not meant to be the end of your daily practice, but only the beginning. As you go about your business, hang onto all the elements of Valsalva Control that you experienced during resonant speech. Remember through the day to:

• Keep a relaxed rectum and an open larynx;

• Breathe with your diaphragm;

• Relax your abdomen as you exhale or speak; and

• "Think phonation," keeping your vocal cords in constant readiness.

From time to time, when others can't hear you, bring your vocal cords together to make a barely audible "aaah" sound. Whenever you get the chance, read aloud or speak to yourself in Adronian.

Approaching Speaking Situations

When you first approach speaking situations, your old attitudes and behavior patterns are likely to re-emerge. Your attempts to relax the Valsalva mechanism may falter. You may need the help of some additional fluency-enhancing methods to control your speech.

Ideally, the need to rely on fluency techniques will diminish as you increase your skills in Valsalva Control. Once you achieve direct control over the Valsalva mechanism, you should be able to talk freely and naturally, without any special methods or restrictions. But this will not come immediately.

In the meantime, we shall suggest a number of techniques that might be used while speaking. They will tie together some of the basic principles of Valsalva Control with several existing fluency methods that may influence the Valsalva mechanism in various ways (as discussed in Chapters 17 and 18).

Three Key Suggestions

It's difficult for anyone to remember more than a few fluency techniques at a time, especially during the stress of actual speaking situations. Therefore, we have boiled down our advice to *three key suggestions*, which should be kept first and foremost in your mind while speaking:

1. Breathe abdominally, relaxing your abdomen as you exhale.

2. Speak each phrase at the same time you relax your abdomen.

3. Concentrate on phonation, prolonging the first syllable of each phrase if necessary.

Because the abdominal muscles are part of the Valsalva mechanism, relaxing the abdomen will tend to relax the entire Valsalva mechanism as well. This will reduce its tendency to interfere with phonation or to cause forceful closures in the mouth or larynx.

Relaxing the abdomen will also prevent a build up of air pressure in the lungs. This will reduce the risk that air pressure will trigger a Valsalva maneuver and cause the mouth or larynx to block airflow.

Concentrating on phonation will help to "tune up" the vocal cords and to relax the laryngeal muscles that perform effort closure. This will improve vocalization, while at the same time relaxing the Valsalva mechanism. Prolongation is a well-known method of emphasizing phonation. It can gradually be reduced and eliminated as you increase your control over the Valsalva mechanism.

To make sure that you relax the Valsalva mechanism whenever you speak, think of speech and phonation as flowing from the relaxation of your abdomen. *Relaxing the abdomen should be the underlying act that controls your speech.* This same act will also control the Valsalva mechanism.

It might be helpful simply to *forget about your mouth* when you speak. Instead, concentrate on relaxing your *abdomen* — and pretend that you are speaking through your *navel.*

No speaking technique should be considered a magical ticket to fluency — *this one included.* Nevertheless, it helped me to start speaking when I was tense and felt that I was going to block. Before answering the telephone, for example, I might take a moment:

- To relax my rectal and abdominal muscles,
- To breathe abdominally a few times, and
- To *think* about speaking as I relaxed my abdomen and exhaled.

After I re-established my coordination in this way, I would pick up the receiver and say "Hello" on the next outward breath, while my abdomen relaxed.

Of course, you don't have to wait for the phone to ring in order to practice this technique. You can do it anytime, anywhere. If you're not in a position to speak aloud, you can practice silently by *imagining* yourself speaking at the same time you are relaxing your abdomen and exhaling. Hopefully, this kind of coordination of speech and abdominal relaxation will eventually become so habitual that you won't have to think about it.

Steps for Speaking

Here is an expanded list of steps to follow during everyday speech. Although most of these suggestions have been around for quite a while, they have been selected and modified for the purposes of Valsalva Control. They are presented chronologically, and not necessarily in the order of their overall importance.

1. Look your listener straight in the eye, and maintain eye contact while speaking.

2. Take a full breath, using the diaphragm, and without holding your breath.

3. Relax your abdomen as you exhale, allowing a soft stream of air to flow naturally, and with-

out force, through your open larynx.

4. As you relax your abdomen, bring your vocal cords gently together and begin speech by prolonging the first syllable. (As previously mentioned, prolongation can be gradually reduced and eliminated as you make progress in Valsalva Control.)

5. Think of your speech as coming from your abdomen as it relaxes. You might even place your hand on your belly while speaking and feel the abdomen go out as you inhale and in as you relax and exhale. Time each phrase with the relaxed inward movement of your abdomen as you exhale.

6. Speak slowly, in short phrases. Don't rush your words, and don't be afraid to pause regularly to take a breath.

7. Focus on phonation and vowels. Pay attention to the music and resonance of your voice. Keep your larynx vibrating as much as possible, linking the words together with the constant hum of phonation. Aim for a relaxed, resonant, mellow, and musical voice. Use variety in your intonation and pitch.

8. Don't avoid. Go ahead and say what you want without substitutions or backtracking. *Don't* go back and repeat previous words in the hope of getting a "running start."

9. Begin initial vowel sounds with a "gentle onset." Instead of blocking the airflow to build up air pressure before saying the vowel, ease into the vowel sound gradually.

10. Use very light pressure in articulating consonants, while always thinking about the vowel sound to come.

Remember that no specific speaking technique is, by itself, a substitute for Valsalva relaxation. If you "try hard" while using any of these methods, you may end up by activating your Valsalva mechanism, totally defeating your purpose.

Handling Blocks

When you feel that you are about to block on a word, don't get upset, don't panic, and — above all — *don't force!* Instead, relax your abdominal muscles to release the block, and let the air flow freely. Begin speaking on the outward flow, as your abdomen relaxes.

Don't fall into the trap of seeing a word as an obstacle that requires force to overcome. Remember that force *never* helps — it only increases the blockage. Instead, recognize the word for what it is: simply a series of movements coordinated with the music of your voice.

Resist your habitual urge to force, struggle, or avoid. Slowly and calmly go right into the movements of the word, one at a time, stretching them out as much as you like. (In the next chapter, we'll talk more about dealing with mental attitudes that contribute to blocks.)

If you find yourself struggling or using avoidance behaviors, *stop immediately!* Continuing to struggle will only reinforce your old patterns of stuttering behavior. Instead, use an approach similar to Van Riper's cancellation technique (previously described in Chapter 21). In our version, you would:

- Pause.
- Recall what you were doing or feeling, and notice how it interfered with your speech.
- Re-establish Valsalva control by relaxing your rectum, breathing abdominally, and relaxing your abdomen as you exhale.
- Then, while relaxing your abdomen and exhaling, repeat *only* the word on which you blocked. (Don't go back and repeat previous words.)

This cancellation method requires vigilance, self-discipline, and the courage to acknowledge and confront your stuttering. Once caught up in struggle or avoidance behavior, a person can momentarily forget that there is any other alternative. I often failed to use cancellation, for fear that it would call attention to my stuttering. Rather than stopping and correcting myself, I would continue to struggle and avoid — all the while trying to pretend that it wasn't really happening. This kind of attitude can be a serious obstacle to change.

As we have repeatedly emphasized, learning to control stuttering is like learning to play a sport or a musical instrument. You must be willing to learn from your mistakes. In the next chapter, we will focus on Rule 6 of the Fluency Cycle, concerning the need to view one's speech objectively and to learn from experience.

CHAPTER 28.

Learning from Experience

CONTROLLING STUTTERING is, of course, not as simple as going through the steps of a recipe. There will be many attitudes and behavior patterns working to sabotage you. These may include not only your attitudes before speaking, but also your mental reaction to the experience of stuttering.

As described in Step 6 of the Valsalva-Stuttering Cycle, persons who stutter may view stuttering as confirming their original belief (in Step 1) that speech is difficult. At the same time, they may also get the false impression that their excessive effort ultimately succeeded in forcing the words out. This may reinforce their tendency to activate the Valsalva mechanism and to use force, avoidance, and other stuttering behavior as ways of overcoming the imagined obstacles to speech.

In place of these detrimental reactions, Rule 6 of the Fluency Cycle suggests the following:

• View your speech objectively, without shame or blame.

• Don't consider speech to be a "test" or stuttering to be a "failure." Instead, learn from *all* your speaking experiences, both fluent and disfluent.

• Don't be fooled into thinking that force, struggle, or avoidance behaviors had anything to do with getting your words out.

• Increase your speaking activities as much as possible, and don't let stuttering spoil the fun of communicating with others.

• Maintain your self-esteem, regardless of fluency.

View Speech Objectively

There is a natural tendency to view one's stuttering in very personal terms. Through the years, stuttering may have acquired deep emotional significance. It may be experienced as a personal failing, a loss of "face," or a sign of unworthiness. One's reactions may include anger, frustration, embarrassment, shame, guilt, and despair.

I grew up feeling I had an obligation to berate and blame myself whenever I stuttered. To some extent, this may have been my way of pre-empting the grownups' disapproval. I would "beat them to the punch" by showing remorse for the "bad" thing I had done. Perhaps I even believed that self-punishment would eventually force me to be fluent. However, it's now clear that this approach is self-defeating. It simply increases one's anxiety and the urge to "try hard" in speaking — thereby perpetuating the Valsalva-Stuttering Cycle and making stuttering worse.

On the opposite side of the same coin is the tactic of **denial**. Because I could not accept my stuttering, I sometimes tried to pretend that it wasn't really happening. This allowed me to feel good about myself for at least a little while. But, sooner or later, I would get seriously stuck on a word, or someone would call attention to my stuttering. Suddenly my fragile self-esteem would collapse, and I'd go back to blaming myself more viciously than ever.

These attitudes and reactions can be serious obstacles to understanding and controlling our stuttering. We must shed our feelings of shame or blame and look at our speech objectively — as if we were scientists studying a natural phenomenon.

Learn from Your Stuttering

As we have previously stated, Valsalva Control is not intended to produce "instant fluency" by artificial means. Instead, it is a gradual process of neurologically reprogramming the Valsalva mechanism to reduce its tendency to interfere with speech. Therefore, you should not expect stuttering to disappear all at once. Stuttering should not be considered a "failure" — either of you or the Valsalva approach. Instead, it should be recognized as an important opportunity for learning.

Before blindly continuing to struggle, pause for a moment to see what you're doing, both physically and mentally. Have your larynx, chest, abdomen, and rectum become tense? Are you holding your breath or building up air pressure in your lungs? Are your vocal cords unprepared to phonate when needed? Are you resorting to avoidance tactics, like fillers, starters, uh's and ah's, word substitutions, etc.?

If so, go back and review the suggestions for Valsalva Control contained in the previous chapter. Perhaps you won't succeed at first; the physical reactions in your Valsalva mechanism may be too strong. Nevertheless, you should at least be *aware* of these reactions. Awareness is the first step in learning to control them.

Also check on your mental attitudes. Are you really following Rule 1 of the Fluency Cycle? Are you looking forward to speaking as an easy and pleasant experience? Or do expect it to be a difficult ordeal in which you must "try hard" to hide your stuttering? It may not be possible for you to change these attitudes on the spot. But again, it will help if you are *aware* of them.

Speaking Is Not a "Test"

Speaking situations should not be viewed as a kind of "test." Such an attitude only increases the urge to try harder to force the words out and thereby activates the Valsalva mechanism. Instead, look forward to speaking with a view toward getting as much satisfaction as possible from communicating with your listener — as well as sensual pleasure from the act of speaking and phonating.

Whenever I felt I had to "prove" I that could say a word fluently, I usually was doomed from the start. On those occasions, I had little success in using any fluency technique (Valsalva Control included). As I reached the moment of truth, I would tense up, my breathing would become spasmodic, my larynx would be unable to phonate, and I would find myself totally blocked. Trying to say the word would become a fixation, charged with increasing fear and frustration. When I eventually gave up, or resorted to word substitution or some other cop-out, I would feel angry with myself and disillusioned with whatever fluency method I had been trying.

Later, when I began noticing what happened during these episodes, I found that I was tense throughout my Valsalva mechanism. I realized that, by viewing speech as a "test," I had already taken the first two steps of the Valsalva-Stuttering Cycle — the anticipation of difficulty and the urge to try hard. As long as I persisted in trying to "prove" that I didn't stutter, I would remain locked in the same old neurological rut that led to Valsalva tuning and blockage.

To get out of this trap, it was first necessary to *abandon the struggle*. I'd have to stop for a moment and remember Rule 1 of the Fluency Cycle — especially its suggestion to *accept the fact that you stutter*. I might even consider using Voluntary Valsalva as a way of "announcing" my stuttering to the listener, thereby ending the suspense. Instead of worrying about fluency, I would focus on my *emotional interaction* with the other person. I would imagine myself communicating in a warm, relaxed, friendly, and pleasurable way.

This demonstrates the paradox that can occur when we "force" ourselves to use a fluency method in an attempt to avoid stuttering. The effort may backfire by increasing stress and triggering the Valsalva-Stuttering Cycle. If this happens, don't be discouraged. Just ease up, continue your daily exercises, and let your Valsalva Control develop gradually.

Responding to Fear and Other Emotions

The more stressful the surrounding circumstances, the more important it is to maintain Valsalva Control. Remember, no law says that you *must* respond to stress by holding your breath and tensing up your Valsalva mechanism. This is just something we learned to do, long ago, because we didn't know any better. Maybe it felt like the "right" thing to do. But in reality, it doesn't score us any points. It just sets us up for stuttering.

As you approach a speaking situation and feel the fear rise up, don't panic! After all, it's just an emotion. Let yourself feel it, without flinching. The real problem is not the fear itself, but the way you have learned to *react* to it. (See Jeffers, 1987.) You can learn a different way.

You can learn to react by *relaxing* rather than tensing the Valsalva mechanism, by breathing abdominally in a relaxed way, with an open larynx, rather than holding your breath and bottling yourself up. Once you have adopted this new way of responding, you will not only be better equipped to deal with the anxiety, but also in a position to speak more fluently.

I learned to do this as a trial lawyer, in order to cope with the highly stressful environment of the courtroom. When confronted with such situations, I now react by relaxing my Valsalva mechanism — which improves my fluency when I need it most.

The same approach can be applied to other emotions, such as anger, when they seem to be messing up your fluency. The idea is to let yourself *feel* the emotion without tensing up your body. Instead, as you focus on the emotion, relax your rectum and abdomen and breath abdominally. This may help you discover that you can *be in touch with disturbing emotions while relaxing your Valsalva mechanism at the same time.* Then go ahead and talk, using the Valsalva Control methods previously described.

Of course, these suggestions are no one-shot cure. Changing your habitual reactions will require a lot of practice and self-discipline (and perhaps the assistance of a group or a therapist). It's not easy to confront one's fears and feelings and to deal with them in a new way. Some people may find this exercise to be emotionally grueling. Nevertheless, it may be an essential step in cutting to the heart of the Valsalva-Stuttering Cycle.

Go Out and Talk

People who have overcome stuttering often say that what helped them most was their willingness to get more involved in things — to become more active and outgoing.

You can start by joining a self-help support group for stutterers, if you haven't already done so. Meet the challenge of participating in discussions and giving talks in front of the group. Many new members are scared to death at first, but in almost no time they feel extremely comfortable. Then keep pushing back the frontiers of your speaking experiences, confronting new situations, even if you aren't fluent. Such opportunities might be found in community projects, religious organizations, amateur theatricals, and public speaking clubs, to name a few examples.

Demosthenes began to argue cases even *before* he practiced with the pebbles. I myself became a lawyer before I became fluent. Likewise, you shouldn't just wait around for fluency to come and change your life. It won't happen. Instead, you've got to go out and get involved, talk, and take risks — whether you stutter or not. *This* is the only real way to gain confidence in speaking.

We should not stake our self-esteem on the shifting sands of fluency. If we are to improve our speech, we must build on firmer ground — beginning with the fundamental qualities of *courage, persistence, and a deeply rooted sense of self-respect.*

General References

JEFFERS, S. *Feel the Fear and Do It Anyway.* New York: Fawcett Columbine, 1987.

WEBSTER, W. G., & POULOS, M. G. *Facilitating Fluency: Transfer Strategies for Adult Stuttering Treatment Programs.* Edmonton, AB: Institute for Stuttering Treatment & Research, 1997 (reformatted and reprinted from 1989 work of the same title originally published by Communication Skill Builders, Tucson, AZ).

CONCLUSION:

A New Outlook on Stuttering

GUIDED BY the Valsalva Hypothesis, we have been able to fit together many pieces of the stuttering puzzle. Where once lay a confusing jumble of seemingly contradictory facts and theories, an understandable picture of stuttering is now emerging. While still hypothetical and incomplete, this vision has the potential to lead us out of the "stutterer's quandary," described in Chapter 2, and to alleviate our frustration over the maddening paradoxes of stuttering. Furthermore, it may lay to rest any stigma, any feelings of guilt or shame, any doubts about our worthiness as human beings.

The Valsalva Perspective

As we have seen, the Valsalva mechanism may play a key role in stuttering behavior. If confused with speech, this normal bodily function might cause excessively forceful closures of the mouth or larynx and delays in phonation — two of the basic symptoms of stuttering. The many other varieties of stuttering behavior (described in Chapter 10) could then be explained as attempts to avoid, postpone, or conceal these underlying blocks.

Our hypothesis suggests why we may instinctively block airflow and build up air pressure in an attempt to force out words as if they were "things." We can now understand why this *feels* like the necessary thing to do — even though it makes fluent speech impossible.

While the Valsalva mechanism is only part of the total picture, it may help us link many of the other pieces together in the proper perspective. Through the Valsalva-Stuttering Cycle, we have seen how the one's activation of the Valsalva mechanism might be prompted by the anticipation that speech will be difficult or that extra effort will be needed. This may explain why stuttering occurs in some situations more than others, and why it usually hits hardest on the most important words.

Other factors may also fit into this picture, insofar as they contribute to the anticipation or perception of difficulty. For example, some stutterers' speech might be affected, to varying degrees, by neurological impairments (either inherited or suffered *in utero* or thereafter) or emotional problems. Even when the initial difficulty is due to a neurological weakness, the Valsalva-Stuttering Cycle may describe the individual's learned *reaction*, which may greatly aggravate the symptoms.

Not every stage of stuttering involves the Valsalva mechanism. As discussed in Chapter 13, a child's earliest disfluencies may arise from a number of factors, such as delays in the neurological development of speaking skills, emotional stress, or excessive demands for good speech. We then saw how the child's effortless, whole-word repetitions might gradually progress into forceful blockages, bringing the Valsalva mechanism into play.

The child — already accustomed to using the Valsalva maneuver when exerting effort or expelling bowel movements — may instinctively assume that words can be forced out in the same way. As noted in Chapter 12, this display of effort could also be the child's way of telling his parents: "You can't punish me for stuttering. Look how *hard* I'm trying to please you!"

Continuation of this behavior during certain critical years of childhood may influence the development of nerve pathways in the brain. The pathways linking speech to the Valsalva mechanism might be strengthened by constant use, while those for fluent speech may remain underdeveloped. In this way, the tendency to involve the Valsalva mechanism in speech would become permanently "wired" into the stutterer's brain.

The Valsalva Hypothesis also suggests new ways of approaching many of stuttering's mysteries. For example:

• The fluency enhancing effects of certain speaking techniques and auditory conditions might be traced to their effect in counteracting various steps in the Valsalva-Stuttering Cycle (as analyzed in Chapters 17 and 18).

• The tremendous predominance of males in the stuttering population might be related, in some degree, to sexual differences in the Valsalva mechanism (as suggested in Chapter 13).

• There may be some connection between certain anomalies found in stutterers' brain function, such as bilateral speech, and their tendency to confuse speech and the Valsalva mechanism (as noted in Chapter 16).

Implications for Stuttering Control

The Valsalva Hypothesis also provides insights that may improve our control of stuttering. In Chapters 19 through 21, we saw how various types of therapy could be explained in terms of their effect on the Valsalva-Stuttering Cycle; how many competing forms of therapy have certain elements in common; and why relapses may occur when stutterers "try hard" to use fluency techniques and thereby activate the Valsalva mechanism.

Our hypothesis views most developmental stutterers as having the basic capacity for reasonably fluent speech. The major problem, in our view, is usually not a *lack* of ability to speak, but rather an *interference* with that ability by the Valsalva mechanism. (Even for the person whose speech is affected by neurological impairments, using the Valsalva mechanism to force the words can only make matters worse.)

Therefore, our approach to fluency does not concentrate on retraining the speech mechanism, but rather on controlling the Valsalva mechanism. Our suggestions for Valsalva Control include both physical and psychological aspects, as seen in the Fluency Cycle. Although we have incorporated a number of fluency methods from the past, they are now intended for the specific purpose of relaxing the Valsalva mechanism and breaking the Valsalva-Stuttering Cycle.

No speaking technique can, by itself, guarantee fluency. However, there is still value in practicing speaking skills. By improving our underlying speaking ability, we can increase our self-confidence and strengthen our nerve pathways for speech. This, in turn, may help to reduce our anticipation of difficulty and our urge to activate the Valsalva mechanism.

One of the practical advantages of Valsalva Control is its compatibility with other forms of stuttering therapy. Therefore, one need not rely exclusively on this approach. Various elements of Valsalva Control can be selected to improve or supplement other treatment programs, and to deal with the tendency to relapse.

Stimulating Further Research

It is truly amazing that researchers have paid so little attention to the Valsalva mechanism, given its potential for explaining so much about stuttering. One reason, I suspect, is that they have viewed it merely in terms of the laryngeal closures that typically occur during an ordinary Valsalva maneuver. Because the larynx does not always close in this fashion during stuttering, researchers may have simply assumed that the Valsalva mechanism was not involved.

In contrast, we have taken a much broader view of the Valsalva mechanism. As we demonstrated in Chapter 6, it can stimulate forceful closures in the *mouth* as well as the larynx. We have also raised the possibility that neurological preparation for a Valsalva maneuver might interfere with the normal prephonatory tuning of the larynx, thereby delaying phonation and interfering with speech.

I recognize that the Valsalva Hypothesis is still only that — a hypothesis — and that considerable scientific research is needed to establish the true role of the Valsalva mechanism in stuttering. As previously suggested, this research might include EMG studies of muscular activity in the Valsalva mechanism during stuttering; testing the effect of Valsalva relaxation on fluency; exploring the neurological relationship between speech and the

Valsalva mechanism; and searching for neurotransmitters or other chemicals that may trigger the Valsalva maneuver.

Because I am not a speech pathologist and don't have access to a speech lab, I can't obtain this data on my own. My only avenue has been to explain my hypothesis and its ramifications as comprehensively as possible, to explore these ideas with other persons who stutter, and to try to stimulate speech pathologists to pursue the necessary research.

Whether or not one accepts my hypothesis, I can see no scientific justification for refusing to investigate the Valsalva mechanism. Researchers have delved into countless aspects of stutterers' behavior and physiology — rarely on the basis of any theory that would explain as much about stuttering as the Valsalva Hypothesis. Unfortunately, it's not likely that the scientific community will undertake this task any time soon, given the fact that research money is scarce and speech scientists already have enough trouble getting their *own* projects funded.

Although the scientists have not yet confirmed the validity of the Valsalva Hypothesis, we who stutter need not wait. We can informally experiment with it ourselves. We can be our own researchers, our own subjects, using our minds, bodies, and speaking experiences as our laboratories. While this approach may not be "scientific," it's all that we have — and all that may really matter.

Educating the Public

Persons who stutter are frequently the victims of ridicule, discrimination, and negative stereotyping. As with many forms of prejudice, the underlying causes may include ignorance and lack of understanding.

The general public has no comprehension of the physiological forces that block a stutterer's speech. Most people cling to the popular notion that stuttering is caused by "nervousness." Studies indicate that this is due to people's tendency to equate stuttering with their own moments of disfluency — which may have been prompted by nervousness, fear, uncertainty, or emotional conflict. They assume that the stutterer is experiencing similar feelings — only more so. Consequently, they may view stutterers as being "nervous," slow, ineffectual, indecisive, or mentally unstable.

Attempts have been made in recent decades to disabuse people of the notion that stuttering is an "emotional problem." In its place, the public has been offered a picture of stuttering that refers instead to possible neurological and hereditary causes. While this view may remove the stigma of mental illness, it may also leave a negative impression, in some minds, that stutterers are hopelessly brain-damaged or inherently defective.

The Valsalva Hypothesis avoids the stigmas that might be associated with both the extreme "psychological" and "neurological" viewpoints by providing an explanation that emphasizes the stutterer's basic normality. We can now talk to people more confidently about stuttering. We need not hem and haw about its mysterious and unknown causes (which may seem potentially sinister to some people). We don't have to tell them that we were psychologically screwed up as children or that we have abnormal fears of speaking, a possible brain deficiency, or vague inherited defects. Now we have a hypothesis that makes things a lot easier. We can honestly tell people:

"No one knows the cause of stuttering for sure, but there is a new hypothesis that seems to explain it as well as anything. Stuttering may be largely due to *a neurological confusion between two basically normal bodily functions* — speech and the Valsalva mechanism. When I anticipate that speaking may be difficult, I may have a tendency to activate the Valsalva mechanism, which is something everybody normally uses to help them exert effort or to force things out of the body."

We might even demonstrate by having our listeners do the hand-pulling exercises described in Chapter 6, to experience how the Valsalva mechanism works. They can then personally feel the pressure in their *own* larynx, lips, and tongue and imagine how this could interfere with their *own* speech. Having experienced the *physiological* force behind stuttering, they may feel less dubious about our mental health and more comfortable about our problem. We can now go on to share a lot more about the stuttering experience.

Overcoming Negative Stereotyping

Research has confirmed that the persons who stutter are subject to negative stereotypes, which have significantly harmed their employment and promotion opportunities. These negative views of persons who stutter are shared by almost all groups studied — students, teachers, employers, parents, even speech-language pathologists. Even worse, studies show that *persons who stutter also believe these stereotypes* — and tend to *behave* accordingly. It seems that people who stutter are not only victims of the stereotype, but they themselves may help to *perpetuate* it.

Ironically, the negative image of stutterers may be made even *worse* by our attempts to avoid or to disguise our stuttering. For example, rather than acknowledging a block, we might pretend that we have forgotten the word, can't decide what to say, or don't know the answer to a question. Or we might engage in inappropriate word substitutions or circumlocutions. While we may think we have fooled people by doing this, we really haven't. We have merely confirmed the stereotype that stutterers are hesitant, indecisive, or stupid.

In terms of listener reaction, research has shown that trying to hide our stuttering is actually the *worst* thing we can do. Studies have shown that listeners have a much more favorable impression of stutterers who acknowledge their stuttering than of stutterers who do not. Listeners also have a more favorable reaction to actual stuttering blocks, repetitions, and prolongations than to the kind of interjections (um's and ah's, etc.) that we often use when we try to avoid stuttering.

Therefore, if we are to break the negative stereotypes, we must accept and acknowledge our stuttering. We must come "out of the closet" and let employers and others know that stuttering is no stigma and nothing to be ashamed of.

Fighting Discrimination

Of the many obstacles faced by people who stutter, perhaps the most costly is *employment discrimination*. I am convinced that this discrimination against stutterers is at least as pervasive as racial or sexual discrimination. In some ways it is even more insidious, because: (1) stutterers are a much smaller minority with less political clout; and (2) many people feel justified in assuming that stuttering is a legitimate job disqualification or a sign of incompetence.

The occurrence and impact of discrimination may vary from person to person depending on a variety of factors — such as the severity of stuttering, the kind of work, and the marketability of the individual's other skills. Some stutterers say that they have never encountered employment discrimination. Many people have achieved success despite their stuttering. Given a chance, people who stutter have distinguished themselves in all walks of life — including business, law, medicine, science, literature, entertainment, and even politics. Nevertheless, for persons not so fortunate, employment discrimination continues to be a problem with serious consequences.

During my 15 years as a National Stuttering Association chapter leader and then as Chair of the NSA's Advocacy Committee, I have heard from stutterers who try to hide their stuttering on the job for fear of being fired, who suffer harassment or unfavorable evaluations by intolerant supervisors, and who have been denied promotions to supervisory positions or jobs that involve speaking or dealing with the public. I personally felt the sting of employment discrimination early in my legal career, when I was openly rejected by firms because of my stuttering, despite my academic qualifications.

Our right to equal opportunity should *not* be conditioned upon our fluency. Every person who stutters should have the right to accept his or her own stuttering — and to insist that employers judge them solely upon their ability to perform the essential requirements of the job in question.

A pretext commonly used by employers to reject stutterers is the job requirement of "excellent oral communications skills." Often this has been invoked simply because the job occasionally involved answering the telephone or speaking to people. Employers must learn that (except in the most severe cases) persons who stutter are capable of adequate — and often very effective — oral communication, regardless of their disfluency. If stuttering disqualifies them from every job that involves some speaking or use of the telephone, they will be excluded from vast areas of the job market — and particularly from the most desirable jobs.

The greatest obstacle to communication comes when people feel compelled to *hide* their stuttering out of fear of reprisal. For employers to demand fluency as the price of one's job only creates a vicious spiral of stress and anxiety that makes stuttering worse.

In fighting stuttering discrimination, we can each be our own best advocates. We can begin by:

• Rooting out our own negative stereotypes and feelings of shame about stuttering;

• Presenting our stuttering in a positive, open, and straightforward way, without trying to hide behind annoying and self-defeating avoidance behaviors; and

• Educating employers and the public about the nature of stuttering, to help them feel more accepting of it, and to show how intolerance only aggravates the situation. The Valsalva Hypothesis might help in this regard.

As a last resort, we may pursue legal remedies to challenge acts of discrimination. In the United States, a number of state and federal statutes now purport to outlaw discrimination against persons with handicaps or disabilities.

The Americans with Disabilities Act of 1990 ("ADA") is a federal statute that bans discrimination "against qualified individuals because of a disability, in regard to job application procedures, hiring, advancement, discharge, compensation, job training, and other terms, conditions, and privileges of employment." It currently applies to employers with 15 or more employees. The Rehabilitation Act of 1973 provides protection for handicapped individuals employed by federal agencies or employers receiving federal funds. Other employers may be covered by various state laws. Each statute has its own specific terms, applicability, and procedures, which must be followed precisely.

I appreciate the fact that many people who stutter dislike being called "handicapped" or "disabled." Of course, *we* know that stuttering need not be a handicap. But the purpose of these laws is to protect us from discrimination by people who aren't so enlightened. To qualify for legal protection, we must therefore be open and "up front" about our stuttering. The worst mistake would be to try to *hide* your stuttering in a way that truly interferes with your job performance (such as by not talking, avoiding the phone, etc.). This might give the employer a legitimate excuse for firing you — even if stuttering itself wouldn't be.

Unfortunately, discrimination cases are usually very hard to win, even for experienced attorneys, so they should not be undertaken haphazardly. As in other disability cases, the threshold question will be whether the individual's stuttering qualifies as a "disability" as defined in the relevant statute. This determination must be made on a case-by-case basis and is subject to many legal technicalities.

Because stuttering is such a complex and misunderstood disorder, stuttering discrimination cases must be carefully planned and prepared in order to avoid potential disaster. My greatest fear is that poorly prepared cases will result in unfavorable judicial opinions, which will then be followed by courts in other cases and seriously damage the rights of all persons who stutter. It would be a tragedy if we allowed the popular prejudices and misconceptions about stuttering to become enshrined as judicial precedent, leaving millions of persons who stutter without legal protection.

A Closing Word

In this book, I have described my own way of understanding and controlling a problem that had tormented me since childhood. With the help of the Valsalva Hypothesis and Valsalva Control, I was finally able to get a handle on stuttering and change my life.

However, I don't claim to have "found the answer" for everyone. Because stuttering is such a personal matter, the only "answer" that really counts must be discovered by each individual who stutters. We must each find our own way "out of the woods."

While seeking to improve our fluency, we must also remember that fluency is *not* the meaning of our existence. As we have seen, the quest for perfect speech is unrealistic, unnecessary, and ultimately self-defeating.

We may never reach the point where we are absolutely fluent all the time. Ingrained in the nerve pathways of our brains, stuttering may linger with us, to one degree or another, throughout our lives.

Nevertheless, we can understand stuttering to the extent that it no longer torments us, and we can control stuttering to the extent that it no longer interferes with our ability to communicate effectively with others. We now have an exciting opportunity to transform our speaking experiences into something far easier and more enjoyable than ever before.

General References

Hurst, M. L., & Cooper, E. B. Employer attitudes toward stuttering. *Journal of Fluency Disorders,* 1983a, 8, 1-12.

Kalinowski, J. S., Lerman, J. W., & Watt, J. A preliminary examination of the perception of self and others in stutterers and nonstutterers. *Journal of Fluency Disorders,* 1987, 14, 127-134.

Lass, N. J., Ruscello, D. M., Schmitt, J. F., Pannbacker, M. D., Orlando, M. B., Dean, K. A., Ruziska, J. C., & Bradshaw, K. H. Teachers' perceptions of stutterers. *Language, Speech. and Hearing Services in Schools,* 1992, 23, 78-81.

Opp, K. L., Hayden, P. A., & Cottrell, G.T. Stuttering and employment: A survey report. Annual Convention of the American Speech. Language, and Hearing Association. Boston, Massachusetts, 1997.

Parry, W. D. Being Your Own Best Advocate & Stuttering as a Disability under the Americans with Disabilities Act of 1990. Anaheim Hills, CA: Nat'l Stuttering Ass'n, 2001.

Parry, W. D. Stuttering and employment discrimination. *Int'l Stuttering Awareness Day 1999 Online Conference, The Stuttering Home Page,* URL: www.mankato.msus.edu/dept/comdis/isad2/papers/parry.html.

White, P. A., & Collins, S. R. C. Stereotype by inference: A possible explanation for the "stutterer" stereotype. *Journal of Speech and Hearing Research,* 1984, 27, 567-570.

Woods, C. L., & Williams, D. E. Traits attributed to stuttering and normally fluent males. *Journal of Speech and Hearing Research,* 1976, 19, 267-278.

Yeakle, M. K., & Cooper, E. B. Teacher perceptions of stuttering. *Journal of Fluency Disorders,* 1986,. 11, 345-359.

Appendices

APPENDIX A:

A Voyage to Adronia

The following story was written as an exercise in Adronian speech for use at a meeting of the Philadelphia Area Chapter of the National Stuttering Project. It is offered here as a whimsical way to become more familiar with the Adronian speech exercise described in Chapter 26.

GOOD NEWS! Our chapter of the NSP has been invited to send a delegation to the Kingdom of Adronia on an all-expense-paid trip. It seems that King Algernon of Adronia recently read an article about stuttering and wants to learn more about this fascinating phenomenon. Adronia is the only country in the world where stuttering does not exist, and the King would like us to teach him about it, and perhaps give a few demonstrations. In return, His Majesty has promised to make a generous donation to the NSP.

Adronia is an island and is reachable only by boat, since it has no airports. During our visit, we will have a chance to investigate whether it is really true that no one stutters in Adronia and, if so, why not.

That's the *good* news.

The *bad* news is that, according to an ancient tradition, only the Adronian language may be spoken within the Kingdom of Adronia. The Adronians are very strict about this. In fact, speaking any language other than Adronian is a capital offense. Violators are immediately spirited away by the Adronian Guards, placed in a catapult, and flung over the castle walls into the royal moat, where they are devoured by the royal crocodiles.

Therefore, in order to assure the safe return of all our members, we are instituting a mandatory crash course in the Adronian language. We are told by the people at Berlitz that it is really easy to learn, and that the words are basically the same as English.

Our chapter was selected for this honor because it is well known that our members are quite adventurous and are always eager to try something new. So let's all give it a try. Remember, you will not be permitted to go on the trip until you are adept at Adronian. (Notice that we didn't say "fluent." You are still free to stutter as much as you like.)

An Introduction to Adronian

Technically, Adronian is not really a separate language, but rather a peculiar dialect of English. The words are the same as in English, with the following differences:

Adronians speak slowly, in short phrases, and every phrase begins with the sound "aa."

Throughout each phrase, the Adronians keep their vocal cords vibrating (phonating) all the time. They never stop making a sound with their voice — even for an instant — until the phrase is completed. This constant phonation sounds something like a drone. Hence the name "Adronian" ("aa" plus "drone").

Lesson One

The Adronian dialect is easy to learn — so easy that even a toddler could do it. To demonstrate this, let us start very simply with the following practice, as we learn gradually to form the words "mommy," "daddy," and "baby." Remember to keep making an unbroken, voiced sound during the entire phrase. Let one sound flow right into the next, without stopping your voice for even an instant. To remind you of this, we have linked the sounds together with dashes.

> Aaaaaaaaa.
> Aaaaaaa-maaa-maaa.
> Aa-maaa-meee.
> Aa-mommy.
>
> Aaaaaaa-daaa-daaa.
> Aa-daaa-deee.
> Aa-daddy.
>
> Aaaaaaa-baaa-baaa.
> Aa-bay-beee.
> Aa-baby.

Well, was that easy or wasn't it? If you were doing it properly, you made a continuous drone of sound, from the beginning of the phrase to the end, without any interruption. When you said the consonants (the *m*, *d*, and *b*), you should have touched the lips or tongue lightly, while continuing to phonate.

Lesson Two

We will now practice building sentences, using words that are almost the same as in our normal English. Say the sentences printed in **bold**. *[The translation is italicized, in brackets.]* There should be no break or pause between "aa" and any of the words in the phrase. One word should flow right into the next, without any interruption whatsoever. To remind you of this, we have linked the words together with dashes. When you come to a slash (/), stop and take a breath, and then start again with "aa" at the beginning of the next phrase.

> *[We are going on a voyage.]*
> **aa-We-are-going/ aa-on-a-voyage.**

(Remember not to interrupt your voice between "aa" and "on." One vowel sound should slide right into the next one.)

> *[Where are we going?]*
> **aa-Where-are-we-going?**
>
> *[Adronia.]*
> **aa-Adronia.**

(Again, there should no hesitation at all between "aa" and "Adronia.")

> *[When do we leave?]*
> **aa-When-do-we-leave?**
>
> *[Now.]*
> **aa-Now.**
>
> *[Bring me my bag.]*
> **aa-Bring-me-my-bag.**
>
> *[Are you ready?]*
> **aa-Are-you-ready?**
>
> *[I am ready.]*
> **aa-I-am-ready.**
>
> *[We are going on a liner.]*
> **aa-We-are-going/ aa-on-a-liner.**
>
> *[The liner is big.]*
> **aa-The-liner-iz-big.**
>
> *[We are going on board.]*
> **aa-We-are-going/ aa-on-board.**
>
> *[The bell rings loudly.]*
> **aa-The-bell-ringz-loudly.**
>
> *[Away we go.]*
> **aa-Away-we-go.**
>
> *[I need a good meal.]*
> **aa-I-need/ aa-a-good-meal.**
>
> *[Where is the galley?]*
> **aa-Where-iz/ aa-the-galley?**
>
> *[Over there.]*
> **aa-Over-there.**
>
> *[Give me a bagel and eggs.]*
> **aa-Give-me/ aa-a-bagel-and-eggz.**
>
> *[Enjoy your meal.]*
> **aa-Enjoy-your-meal.**
>
> *[The waves are bigger now.]*
> **aa-The-wavez/ aa-are-bigger-now.**

[My meal is moving around.]
aa-My-meal/ aa-iz-moving-around.

[Where is the railing?]
aa-Where-iz-the-railing?

[There is the railing.]
aa-There-iz-the-railing.

[I am running there now.]
aa-I-am-running/ aa-there-now.

[I am leaning over the railing.]
aa-I-am-leaning/ aa-over-the-railing.

[Goodbye, bagel and eggs.]
aa-Goodbye,/ aa-bagel-and-eggz.

A Word About Voiced and Unvoiced Consonants

The previous lesson was limited strictly to words that would sound the same in both English and Adronian. You will notice that all of the sounds in those words were voiced sounds. The vocal cords never had to stop vibrating (phonating) from the beginning of a phrase to its end. In English, however, some consonants are voiced and some are unvoiced. (See the table in Chapter 26, which shows a list of unvoiced consonants and the corresponding voiced consonants which replace them.)

In Adronian, the voice never stops until the end of a phrase. As a result, every unvoiced consonant in English is replaced by its corresponding *voiced* consonant.

"Wait a minute!" you might be thinking. "All of this is too complicated to remember. Isn't there an easier way?"

Indeed there is. All you need to know is this: Your mouth moves exactly the same as it does when you say the English words, and all the vowels are the same. The only difference is that your vocal cords keep vibrating all the time during each phrase. Once you learn to keep your vocal cords phonating all the time, while you move your mouth the usual way, Adronian comes automatically.

Lesson Three

We now practice sentences in which the unvoiced consonants in English are transformed into their corresponding voiced consonants in Adronian. Say the sentences as they are written in bold. Remember: Move your mouth exactly as you do in English, while constantly phonating throughout each phrase.

[Are you feeling better now?]
aa-Are-you-veeling/ aa-bedder-now?

[Yes, thank you.]
aa-Yez,/ aa-thang-you.

(Note that the "th" in "thank" is changed to a voiced sound.)

[Let's play a game.]
aa-Led'z-blay-a-game.

[What would you like to play?]
aa-Whad-would-you/ aa-lieg-do-blay?

[Let's play ping pong.]
aa-Led'z-blay/ aa-bing-bong.

[Sorry, there are no ping pong paddles.]
aa-Zorry, aa-there-are-no/
aa-bing-bong-baddlez.

[Anyone for tennis?]
aa-Anyone-vor-denniz?

[Sorry, there is no tennis court.]
aa-Zorry,/ aa-there-iz-no/ aa-denniz-gourd.

[Let's swim in the swimming pool.]
aa-Led'z-zwim/ aa-in-the-zwimming-bool.

[Sorry, there is no swimming pool.]
aa-Zorry,/ aa-there-iz-no/ aa-zwimming-bool.

[Then what can we do on this tub?]
aa-Then-whad-gan-we-do/ aa-on-thiz-dub?

[We can play shuffle board.]
aa-We-gan-blay/ aa-zhuvvle-board.

[I can see this will be a long trip.]
aa-I-gan-zee/ aa-thiz-will-be/ aa-a-long-drib.

Lesson Four

Now let's practice translating some more familiar things into Adronian.

Figure out how to say the following in Adronian, and practice each at least 5 times:
- Your name;
- Your address;
- Your telephone number;
- Names of your friends, spouse, or family members.

Recite "A Stutterer's Declaration" in Adronian, filling in your name:

aa-A-Zdudderer'z-Deglarazion

[My name is _____.]
aa-My-name-iz/ aa-_____.

[I am a person who stutters.]
aa-I-am-a-berzon/ aa-oo-zdudderz.

[I can live with that, and so can you.]
aa-I-gan-live-with-thad,/ aa-and-zo-gan-you.

[I'm not afraid to stutter,]
aa-I'm-nod-avraid-do-zdudder,/

[and I'm not afraid to change,]
aa-and-I'm-nod-avraid-do-jange,

[As every day I learn more and more control.]
aa-Az-every-day/ aa-I-learn-more-and-more/ aa-gondrol.

A Few Words About the Adronians

Before we set foot in the Kingdom of Adronia, it is important to know something about the peculiar habits and manners of the Adronian people.

Most Adronians are very leisurely and easy-going. They talk slowly, walk slowly, work slowly. (That's one of the reasons they don't have an airport; no one's in a hurry to get anywhere.) But despite this, they manage to move steadily along. They look people right in the eye, say what has to be said, and do what has to be done.

Adronians consider it rude to talk fast, to rush people, or to interrupt. It is also rude not to maintain eye contact during conversation. In fact, most Andronians don't have telephones, because they would rather talk to people face-to-face.

So, when you approach an Adronian, remember: Be friendly, maintain eye contact, and take your time. They like to talk and they like to listen. You might as well relax and enjoy it also.

Lesson Five

Next we practice speaking in specific kinds of situations that might arise after we arrive in Adronia. In each situation, one person will play the part of the Adronian and another person will play the part of the Visitor. The following dialogues are offered only as examples to get you started. Improvise your own conversations in Adronian.

Whenever someone forgets to speak Adronian, they should be promptly reminded by others in the group. This can be done by shouting "aa-Boing!" to symbolize the catapult that flings violators to the crocodiles.

Going Through Customs

OFFICER: *[Welcome to Adronia.]*
aa-Welgome-do-Adronia./

[What is your name?]
aa-Whad-iz-your-name?

VISITOR: *[My name is: _____.]*
aa-My-name-iz/ aa-_____.

OFFICER: *[May I please see your passport?]*
aa-May-I-bleaze/ aa-zee-your-bazzbord?

VISITOR: *[Here is my passport.]*
aa-Eer-iz-my-bazzbord./

[The picture really doesn't do me justice.]
aa-The-bigjure-really-doezn'd/aa-do-me-juzdiz.

OFFICER: *[Please open your suitcase.]*
aa-Bleaze-oben-your-zoodgaze.

VISITOR: *[Certainly.]*

aa-Zerdainly./

[I have the key around here somewhere.]
aa-I-ave-the-gey/ aa-around-eer-zomewhere.

OFFICER: [Have you anything to declare?]
aa-Ave-you-anything/ aa-do-deglare?

VISITOR: [Yes. I am a person who stutters.]
aa-Yez./ aa-I-am-a-berzon-oo-zdudderz./

[I can live with that, and so can you.]
aa-I-gan-live-with-thad,/ aa-and-zo-gan-you.

Taking the Taxi

DRIVER: [Where to?]
aa-Where-do?

VISITOR: [The Hotel Adronia.]
aa-The-Odel-Adronia.

DRIVER: [Of course.]
aa-Ov-gourze./

That's where all the visitors stay.]
aa-Thad'z-where/ aa-all-the-vizidorz-zday.

VISITOR: [Why? Is it the best hotel in A-dronia?]
aa-Why?/ aa-Iz-id-the-bezd-odel/ aa-in-Adronia?

DRIVER: [No. It's the only hotel.]
aa-No./ aa-Id'z-the-*only*-odel.

VISITOR: [I see.]
aa-I-zee.

DRIVER: [What country are you from?]
aa-Whad-goundry-are-you-vrom?

VISITOR: [The United States.]
aa-The-Unided-Zdaidz.

DRIVER: [How long are you staying?]
aa-Ow-long-are-you-zdaying?

VISITOR: [That depends on the crocodiles.]
aa-Thad-debendz/ aa-on-the-grogodielz.

DRIVER: [Don't worry.]
aa-Don'd-worry./

[You are speaking the language fine.]
aa-You-are-zbeaging/ aa-the-language-vine.

VISITOR: [I hate to sound impatient, but can't this taxi go any faster?]
aa-I-ade-do-zound-imbaziend,/ aa-bud-gan'd-thiz-dagzi/ aa-go-any-vazder?

DRIVER: [No, but it can go a lot slower.]
aa-No,/ aa-bud-id-gan-go/ aa-a-lod-zlower.

VISITOR: [What would you do if there was an emergency?]
aa-Whad-would-you-do/ aa-iv-there-waz/ aa-an-emergenzy?

DRIVER: [Personally, I'd get out of the cab and walk.]
aa-Berzonally,/ aa-I'd-ged-oud-ov-the-gab/ aa-and-wogg.

Looking for a Telephone

VISITOR: [Where is the telephone?]
aa-Where-iz-the-delevone?

NATIVE: [We have no telephone.]
aa-We-ave-no-delevone.

VISITOR: [Then how can I "reach out and touch someone"?]
aa-Then-ow-gan-I/ "aa-reaj-oud-and-douj-zomeone"?

NATIVE: [You'll have to do it in person.]
aa-You'll-ave-do-do-it/ aa-in-berzon./

[But in the meantime, please keep your hands to yourself.]
aa-But-in-the-meandime,/ aa-bleaze-geeb-your-andz/ aa-do-yourzelv.

At the Restaurant

VISITOR: [Waiter! I just found a dead mouse in my soup.]
aa-Waider!/ aa-I-juzd-vound-a-dead-mouze/ aa-in-my-zoub.

WAITER: [Well, of course.]
aa-Well-ov-gourze./

[Did you expect to find a live one?]
aa-Did-you-exbegd-do-vind/ aa-a-live-one?

VISITOR: [I'm not hungry any more.]
aa-I'm-nod-ungry-any-more./

[Would you please just bring me a cup of coffee.]
aa-Would-you-bleaze-juzd-bring-me/
aa-a-gub-ov-govvee.

WAITER: [Certainly. How would you like your coffee?]
aa-Zerdainly./
aa-Ow-would-you-lieg/ aa-your-govvee?

VISITOR: [Without cream, please.]
aa-Withoud-gream-bleaze.

WAITER: [We don't have any cream.]
aa-We-don'd-ave-any-gream.

VISITOR: [All right, then. I'll have it without milk.]
aa-All-right-then./ aa-I'll-ave-id-withoud-milg.

Looking for the Bathroom

VISITOR: [Where is the rest room?]
aa-Where-iz-the-rezd-room?

NATIVE: [In Adronia, we rest in every room.]
aa-In-Adronia,/ aa-we-rezd-in-every-room.

VISITOR: [I mean, where is the toilet?]
aa-I-mean,/ aa-where-iz-the-doiledd?

NATIVE: [In that little shed way out back.]
aa-In-thad-liddle-zhed/ aa-way-oud-bag.

VISITOR: [You mean you make people go all the way across the back yard to use the toilet?]
aa-You-mean-you-maeg-beoble/
aa-go-all-the-way/ aa-agrozz-the-bag-yard/
aa-do-use-the-doiledd?

NATIVE: [In Adronia, that's the only chance we get to see people run.]
aa-In-Adronia,/
aa-thad'z-the-only-janze-we-ged/
aa-do-zee-beoble-run.

A Medical Riddle

QUESTION: [What is the first thing Adronians do when they go to the doctor?]
aa-Whad-iz-the-virzd-thing/ aa-Adronians-do/
aa-when-they-go-do-the-dogdor?

ANSWER: [They open their mouths and say "Aa."]
aa-They-oben-their-mouthz/ aa-and-zay-"Aa."

Lesson Six

As in the learning of any language or other skill, proficiency at Adronian requires practice, practice, and practice. Don't expect to get away easy. You should practice Adronian at home for about a half hour every day until it becomes so habitual that it is second nature to you.

Once you master the technique, the result will be instant Adronian. You will be able to say anything in Adronian, without thinking twice about it. Once you feel comfortable reading in Adronian, you may gradually speak in longer phrases. You may even discover that reading aloud in Adronian is very relaxing. Best of all, you will be able to stop worrying about the crocodiles.

Whenever you are alone and no one can hear, start talking Adronian again. For example, when driving alone in an automobile, you can read license plates, road signs, and billboards out loud in Adronian. Nobody has to know. Of course, there may be some situations in which you simply don't care if another person hears you talking Adronian. For example, when a solicitor calls you on the telephone. In that case, Adronian may be a perfect way to get him to hang up.

APPENDIX B:

Organizations and Resources for Stuttering Information and Self-Help

This list is by no means complete. It represents only a few examples of organizations and other resources operating in the United States, Canada, and around the world. (Although the following information is believed to be current as of this printing, it is subject to change at any time.)

United States

National Stuttering Association
119 W. 40th Street, 14th Floor
New York, NY 10018
Newsletter: *Letting Go*
Telephone: 1-800-WE STUTTER
e-mail: info@WeStutter.org
Website: www.WeStutter.org

American Speech-Language-Hearing Association
10801 Rockville Pike
Rockville, MD 20852
Telephone: 1-800-638-8255
Website: www.asha.org

Friends
Website: www.friendswhostutter.org

Passing Twice: GLB&T People Who Stutter
Website: www.passingtwice.com

Speak Easy International Foundation, Inc.
233 Concord Drive, Paramus, NJ 07652
Newsletter: *The Speak Easy Newsletter*

Stuttering Foundation of America
P.O. Box 11749
Memphis, TN 38111-0749
Telephone: 1-800-992-9392
Newsletter: *SFA Newsletter*
Website: www.stuttersfa.org

The Stuttering Home Page
Website: www.stutteringhomepage.com

Canada

Association des Begues du Canada, Inc.
7801 Rue Ste-Claire
Montreal, Quebec H1L 1V8 Canada

Canadian Association for People Who Stutter
P.O. Box 444, Branch NDG
Montreal QC H4A 3P8, Canada
Website: www.webcon.net/~caps/

Speak Easy, Inc.
95 Evergreen Avenue
Saint John, NB E2N 1H4, Canada
Website: www.speakeasycanada.com

Argentina

Asociacion Argentina de Tartamudez
Website: www.aat.org.ar

Australia

Australian Speak Easy Association Inc.
Website: www.speakeasy.org.au

Austria

Oesterreichische Selbsthilfe-Initiative Stottern
Website: www.stotternetz.at

Belgium

Belgium Stuttering Association
Website: www.stotteren.be

Denmark

Foreningen for Stammere i Danmark (FSD)
Website: www.fsd.dk

France

Association Parole-Begaiement (A.P.B.)
Website: www.begaiement.org

Germany

Bundesvereinigung Stottererer-Selbsthilfe e.V.
Gereonswall 112, D-50670 Köln, Germany
Website: www.bvss.de/

India

Fluency Club
c/o J. C. Nigam
35-C Pocket I/MayurVihar-Phase-I
Delhi-110091, India

International

European League of Stuttering Associations
Website: www.elsa.info
See website for list of member organizations.

International Fluency Association
Website: www.theifa.org

International Stuttering Association
Website: www.stutterisa.org
See website for list of member organizations.

Ireland

Irish Stammering Association
Carmichael House, North Brunswick Street
Dublin 7, Ireland

Israel

AMBI - Israeli Stuttering Association
Website: www.ambi.org.il

Japan

Japan Stuttering Project
Shinji Ito c/o Kazue Shinji
17-3, Monamiogi-cho, Kamigamo,
Kita-ku, Kyoto 603, Japan

The Netherlands

Nederlands Stottervereniging "Demosthenes"
Postbox 119, NL-3500 AC Utrecht, Netherlands
Website: www.stotteren.nl/

New Zealand

New Zealand Speak Easy Association, Inc.
924A Papamoa Beach Road
Papmoa 3003, New Zealand
Website: www.shopzone.co.nz/speakeasy

Norway

NIFS
Postboks 4568, Nydalen 0404, Oslo, Norway
Website: www.stamming.no

South Africa

Speak Easy Stuttering Association
Website: www.ix.co.za/speakeasy/

Sweden

SSR - Swedish Stuttering Association
c/o Anita S. Blom
Vättlösa, Källåker, S-533 91 Götene, Sweden
Website: www.stamning.se

United Kingdom

The British Stammering Association
15 Old Ford Road, London E2 9PJ England
Newsletter: *Speaking Out*
Website: www.stammering.org

The Author's Website:

The Valsalva Stuttering Network
www.valsalva.org

Bibliography

ADAMS, M. R. A physiologic and aerodynamic interpretation of fluent and stuttered speech. *Journal of Fluency Disorders,* 1974, 1, 35-47.

ADAMS, M. R. & HUTCHINSON, J. The effects of three levels of auditory masking on selected vocal characteristics and the frequency of disfluency of adult stutterers. *Journal of Speech and Hearing Research,* 1974, 17, 682-688,

ADAMS, M. R., & REIS, R. The influence of the onset of phonation on the frequency of stuttering. *Journal of Speech and Hearing Research,* 1971, 14, 639-644.

ADAMS, M. R., & REIS, R. The influence of the onset of phonation on the frequency of stuttering: A replication and re-evaluation. *Journal of Speech and Hearing Research,* 1974, 17, 752754.

AMBROSE, N. G., COX, N. J., & YAIRI, E. The genetic basis of persistence and recovery in stuttering. *Journal of Speech, Language and Hearing Research,* 1997, 40, 567-80.

ANDREWS, G., CRAIG, A., FEYER, A., HODDINOTT, S., HOWIE, P., & NEILSON, M. Stuttering: a review of research findings and theories circa 1982. *Journal of Speech and Hearing Disorders,* 1983, 48, 226-246.

ARDRAM, G. M., & KEMP, F. H. The mechanism of the larynx: II. The epiglottis and closure of the larynx. *British Journal of Radiology,* 1967, 40, 372-389.

ARMSON, J., & STUART, A. Effect of extended exposure to frequency-altered feedback on stuttering during reading and monologue. *Journal of Speech, Language and Hearing Research,* 1998, 41, 479-490.

BAKKER, K. & BRUTTEN, G. A comparative investigation of the laryngeal premotor, adjustment, and reaction times of stutterers and nonstutterers. *Journal of Speech and Hearing Research,* 1989, 32, 239-244.

BAKKER, K. & BRUTTEN, G. Speech-related reaction times of stutterers and nonstutterers: diagnostic implications. *Journal of Speech and Hearing Disorders,* 1990, 55, 295-299.

BEATON, A. *Left Side, Right Side: A Review of Laterality Research.* New Haven: Yale University Press, 1985.

BLOODSTEIN, O. *A Handbook on Stuttering.* 5th ed. San Diego: Singular Publishing Group, 1995.

BLOODSTEIN, O. *Stuttering: The Search for a Cause and Cure.* Needham Heights, MA: Allyn & Bacon, 1993.

BOBERG, E. Relapse and outcome. *Stuttering Then and Now* (edited by Shames, G.H., & Rubin, H.). Columbus, OH: Charles E. Merrill Publishing Co., 1986, 501-513.

BOBERG, E., EDITOR. *Neuropsychology of Stuttering.* Edmonton, Alberta: University of Alberta Press, 1993.

BOBERG, E., HOWIE, P., & WOODS, L. Maintenance of fluency: a review. *Stuttering Then and Now* (edited by Shames, G.H., & Rubin, H.). Columbus, OH: Charles E. Merrill Publishing Co., 1986, 489-500.

BOBRICK, B. *Knotted Tongues.* New York: Simon & Schuster, 1995.

BORDEN, G. J., BAER, T., & KENNEY, M. K. Onset of voicing in stuttered and fluent utterances. *Journal of Speech and Hearing Research,* 1985, 28, 363-372.

BRADY, J. P. Alprazolam, citalopram, and clomipramine for stuttering. Stuttering Foundation of America. URL: www.stuttersfa.org/Research/drugther.htm.

BRADY, J. P. The pharmacology of stuttering: a critical review. *Am. J. Psychiatry,* 1991, 148, 1309-1316.

BRAUN, A. R., VARGA, M., STAGER, S., SCHULZ, G., SELBIE, S., MAISOG, J. M., CARSON, R. E., & LUDLOW, C. L. Altered patterns of cerebral activity during speech and language production in developmental stuttering. *Brain,* 1997, 120, 761-784.

BROOKS, V. B. *The Neural Basis of Motor Control.* New York: Oxford University Press, 1986.

BURNS, D. & BRADY, J. P. Stuttering and speech disorders. *Psychiatric Clinics of North America,* 1978, 1, 335-348.

CARLISLE, J. A. *Tangled Tongue.* Reading, MA: Addison-Wesley Publishing Co., 1985.

CARLSON, A. J., JOHNSON, V., & CAVERT, H. M. *The Machinery of the Body.* Chicago: University of Chicago Press, 1961.

CIPOLOTTI, L., BISIACCHI, P. S., DENES, G., & GALLO, A. Acquired stuttering: a motor programming disorder? *Eur. Neurology,* 1988, 28, 321-325.

CONTURE, E. G. Childhood stuttering: what is it and who does it? *Research Needs in Stuttering: Roadblocks and Future Directions. ASHA Reports,* 1990, 18, 2-14.

CONTURE, E. G., MCCALL, G., & BREWER, D. W. Laryngeal behavior during stuttering. *Journal of Speech and Hearing Research,* 1977, 20, 661-668.

CONTURE, E. G., SCHWARTZ, H. D., & BREWER, D. W. Laryngeal behavior during stuttering: a further study. *Journal of Speech and Hearing Research,* 1985, 28, 233-240.

COOPER, E. B. *Understanding Stuttering: Information for Parents* (rev. ed.). Chicago: National Easter Seal Society, 1990.

DENES, P. B. & PINSON, E. N. *The Speech Chain.* New York: W. H. Freeman & Co., 1993.

DEWAR, A., DEWAR, A. D., AUSTIN, W. T. S., & BRASH, H. M. The long term use of an automatically triggered auditory feedback masking device in the treatment of stammering. *British Journal of Disorders of Communication,* Winter 1979-1980, 14, 3, 219-229.

DICKSON, D. R., & MAUE-DICKSON, W. *Anatomical and Physiological Bases of Speech.* Boston: Little, Brown & Co., 1982.

DIMOND, S. J. *Neuropsychology.* London: Butterworths, 1980.

DE NIL, L. Some thoughts on the multidimensional nature of stuttering from a neurophysiological perspective. *Int'l Stuttering Awareness Day 1998 Online Conference, The Stuttering Home Page,* URL: www.mankato.msus.edu/dept/comdis/isad/papers/denil.html.

DRAYNA, D., KILSHAW, J., & KELLY, J. The sex ratio in familial persistent stuttering. *Am. J. Human Genetics,* 1999, 65, 1473-75.

FARBER, S. *Identical Twins Reared Apart: A Reanalysis.* New York: Basic Books (1981).

FINK, B. R. The curse of Adam: Effort closure of the larynx. *Anesthesiology,* 1973, 39, 325-327.

FINK, B. R. *The Human Larynx: A Functional Study.* New York: Raven Press, 1975.

FINK, B. R., & DEMAREST, R. *Laryngeal Biomechanics.* Cambridge, Mass: Harvard University Press, 1978.

FOUNDAS, A. L. Are the brains of people who stutter different? Stuttering Foundation of America website: www.stuttersfa.org/Research/foundas.htm.

FOX, P. T., INGHAM, R. J., INGHAM, J. C., HIRSCH, T. B., DOWNS, J. H., MARTIN, C., JERABEK, P., GLASS, T., & LANCASTER, J. L. A PET study of the neural systems of stuttering. *Nature,* 1996, 382, 158-162.

FRASER, M. *Self-Therapy for the Stutterer.* 7th ed. Memphis, TN: Speech Foundation of America, 1990.

FREEMAN, J., & USHIJIMA, T. Laryngeal muscle activity during stuttering. *Journal of Speech and Hearing Research,* 1978, 21, 538-561.

FREEMAN, J., USHIJIMA, T., & HIROSE, H. Reply to Schwartz's "The core of the stuttering block". *Journal of Speech and Hearing Disorders,* 1975, 40, 137-139.

FREUND, H. *Psychopathology and the Problems of Stuttering.* Springfield, Ill.: Charles C. Thomas, 1966.

FROESCHELS, E. New viewpoints on stuttering. *Folia Phoniatrica,* 1961, 13, 187-201.

GLAUBER, I. P. Dynamic therapy for the stutterer. *Specialized Techniques in Psychotherapy.* New York: Grove Press, 1952, 207-238.

GOLDSMITH, M. F. Brain studies may alter long-held concepts about likely causes of some voice disorders. *Journal of American Medical Ass'n,* 1989, 261, 964-965.

GRAY, H. *Anatomy of the Human Body.* Philadelphia: Lea & Febiger, 1959.

HARRISON, J. C. *How To Conquer Your Fears of Speaking Before People.* 5th ed. Anaheim Hills, CA: Nat'l Stuttering Ass'n, 1999.

HARRISON, J. C. Why talking is easier when you are "being" someone else. *How To Conquer Your Fears of Speaking Before People.* 5th ed. Anaheim Hills, CA: Nat'l Stuttering Ass'n, 1999.

HARRISON, J. C. Developing a new paradigm for stuttering. *How To Conquer Your Fears of Speaking Before People.* 5th ed. Anaheim Hills, CA: Nat'l Stuttering Ass'n, 1999.

HELM, N. A., BUTLER, R. B., & BENSON, D. F. Acquired stuttering. *Neurology,* 1978, 28, 1159-1165.

HOLE, J. W. *Human Anatomy and Physiology.* Dubuque, Iowa: Wm. C. Brown Co., 1981.

HOOPER, J. & DICK, T. *The Three-Pound Universe.* New York: MacMillan Publishing Co., 1986.

HURST, M. L., & COOPER, E. B. Employer attitudes toward stuttering. *Journal of Fluency Disorders,* 1983a, 8, 1-12.

JACOBSON, E. *Self-Operations Control.* Philadelphia: J.B. Lippincott Co., 1964.

JEFFERS, S. *Feel the Fear and Do It Anyway.* New York: Fawcett Columbine, 1987.

JEZER, M. *Stuttering: A Life Bound Up in Words.* New York: Basic Books, 1997.

JOHNSON, W., ET AL. *The Onset of Stuttering.* Minneapolis: University of Michigan Press, 1959.

JOHNSON, W., ET AL. A study of the onset and development of stuttering. *Stuttering Then and Now* (edited by Shames, G.H., & Rubin, H.). Columbus, OH: Charles E. Merrill Publishing Co., 1986, 125-129.

JONES, R. K. Observations on stammering after localized cerebral injury. *J. Neurology, Neurosurgery & Psychiatry,* 1966, 29, 192-195.

JONES, R. K. Dyspraxic ambiphasia: a neurophysiologic theory of stammering.

KALINOWSKI, J. S., LERMAN, J. W., & WATT, J. A preliminary examination of the perception of self and others in stutterers and nonstutterers. *Journal of Fluency Disorders*, 1987, 14, 127-134.

KEHOE, T. D. *Stuttering: Science, Therapy & Practice.* Boulder, CO: Casa Futura Technologies, 1999.

KENT, R. D. Facts about stuttering: neuropsychologic perspectives. *Journal of Speech and Hearing Disorders*, 1983, 48, 249-255.

KENYON, E. The etiology of stammering: The psychophysiologic facts which concern the production of speech sounds and of stammering. *Journal of Speech and Hearing Disorders*, 1943, 8, 337-348.

LADEFOGED, P. Linguistic aspects of respiratory phenomena. *Annals of New York Academy of Sciences*, 1968, 155, 141-151.

LASS, N. J., RUSCELLO, D. M., SCHMITT, J. F., PANNBACKER, M. D., ORLANDO, M. B., DEAN, K. A., RUZISKA, J. C., & BRADSHAW, K. H. Teachers' perceptions of stutterers. *Language, Speech, and Hearing Services in Schools*, 1992, 23, 78-81.

LASTOVKA, M. The monosynaptic spinal cord reflex activity changes in stuttering. *Folia Phoniatrica*, 1970, 22, 129-138.

LASTOVKA, M. Influence of some psychopharmaca on the increase of the amplitude of electrically induced monosynaptic spinal cord reflex during the paroxysm of stuttering: I. effect of diazepam. *Folia Phoniatrica*, 1979, 31, 15-20.

LASTOVKA, M. Influence of some psychopharmaca on the increase of the amplitude of electrically induced monosynaptic spinal cord reflex during the paroxysm of stuttering: II. effect of chlorpromazine. *Folia Phoniatrica*, 1979, 31, 21-26.

LEE, B. S., MCGOUGH, W. E., & PEINS, M. A. A new method for stuttering therapy. *Folia Phoniatrica*, 1973, 25, 186-195.

LOVE, R. J. & WEBB, W. G. *Neurology for the Speech-Language Pathologist.* Stoneham, MA: Butterworth, 1986.

MAGUIRE, G. A., GOTTSCHALK, L. A., RILEY, G. D., FRANKLIN, D. L., BECHTEL, R. J., & ASHURST, J. Stuttering: neuropsychiatric features measured by content analysis of speech and the effect of risperidone on stuttering severity. *Compr. Psychiatry*, 1999, 4, 308-14.

MALLARD, A. R., HICKS, D. M., & RIGGS, D. E. A comparison of stutterers and nonstutterers in a task of controlled voice onset. *Journal of Speech and Hearing Research*, 1982, 25, 287-290.

MALTZ, M. *Psycho-Cybernetics.* Hollywood, CA: Wilshire Book Co., 1960.

MATEER, C. A. Neural bases of language. *Neuropsychology of Stuttering* (edited by Boberg, E.). Edmonton, Alberta: University of Alberta Press, 1993, 1-24.

MCCALL, GERALD N. & RABUZZI, D. D. Reflex contraction of middle-ear muscles secondary to stimulation of laryngeal nerves. *Journal of Speech and Hearing Research*, 1973, 16, 56-61.

MOORE, W. H. Pathophysiology of stuttering: cerebral activation differences in stutters vs. nonstutterers. *Research Needs in Stuttering: Roadblocks and Future Directions. ASHA Reports*, 1990, 18, 72-80.

MOORE, W. H. Hemispheric processing research. *Neuropsychology of Stuttering* (edited by Boberg, E.). Edmonton, Alberta: University of Alberta Press, 1993, 39-53.

MURRAY, F. P. *A Stutterer's Story.* Memphis, TN: Stuttering Foundation of America, 1991.

MURRAY, F. P. Commentary. *The Speak Easy Newsletter* (Paramus, NJ), Spring 1992, 12, 1, p.6.

NISHIMORA, R. A. & TAJIK, A. J. The Valsalva maneuver and response revisited. *Mayo Clinic Proceedings*, 1986, 61, 211-217.

NOBACK, C. R., STROMINGER, N.L., & DEMAREST, R. J. *The Human Nervous System: Introduction and Review.* 4th ed. New York: McGraw-Hill Book Co., 1991.

OPP, K. L., HAYDEN, P. A., & COTTRELL, G.T. Stuttering and employment: A survey report. Annual Convention of the American Speech, Language, and Hearing Association. Boston, Massachusetts, 1997.

PARRY, W. D. Finding my way out of the woods. *Letting Go*, Jan. 1985a, 5, 1, pp. 6-7.

PARRY, W. D. Stuttering and employment discrimination. *Int'l Stuttering Awareness Day 1999 Online Conference, The Stuttering Home Page*, URL: www.mankato.msus.edu/dept/comdis/isad2/papers/parry.html.

PARRY, W. D. Stuttering and the Valsalva mechanism: a hypothesis in need of investigation. *Journal of Fluency Disorders*, 1985b, 10, 317-324.

PAULS, D. L. A review of the evidence for genetic factors in stuttering. *Research Needs in Stuttering: Roadblocks and Future Directions. ASHA Reports*, 1990, 18, 34-38.

PERKINS, W. H. Replacement of stuttering with normal speech: II. Clinical procedures. *Journal of Speech and Hearing Disorders*, 1973, 38, 295-303.

PERKINS, W. H. The problem of definition: commentary on "stuttering." *Journal of Speech and Hearing Disorders*, 1983, 48, 246-249.

PERKINS, W. H. Do fluency controls ever promote automatic fluency? *American Journal of Speech-Language Pathology*. Jan. 1992.

PERKINS, W., RUDAS, J., JOHNSON, L., & BELL, J.

Stuttering: discoordination of phonation with articulation and respiration. *Journal of Speech and Hearing Research,* 1976, 19, 509-522.

PETERS, H. F. M. & BOVES, L. Coordination of aerodynamic and phonatory processes in fluent speech utterances of stutterers. *Journal of Speech and Hearing Research,* 1988, 31, 352-361.

PETERS, T. J., & GUITAR, B. *Stuttering: An Integrated Approach to Its Nature and Treatment.* Baltimore: Williams & Wilkins, 1991.

PETERSDORF, R. G., ET AL. *Harrison's Principles of Internal Medicine.* New York: McGraw-Hill Book Co., 1983.

REED, S. Susan Reed's keynote speech reviewed the format of CSA. *Speak Easy Newsletter* (Paramus, NJ), Winter 1990, 10, 4, 5-6.

REICH, A., TILL, J., & GOLDSMITH, H. Laryngeal and manual reaction times of stuttering and nonstuttering adults. *Journal of Speech and Hearing Research,* 1981, 24, 192-196.

ROSENFIELD, D. B. Stuttering. *Current Problems in Pediatrics,* 1982, 12, No. 8.

ROSENFIELD, D. B. Stuttering and cerebral ischemia. *New England Journal of Medicine,* 1972, 287, 991.

ROSENFIELD, D. B., MILLER, S. D., & FELTOVICH, M. Brain damage causing stuttering. *Transactions of the American Neurological Ass'n,* 1980, 105, 181-183.

SCHWARTZ, M. The core of the stuttering block. *Journal of Speech and Hearing Disorders,* 1974, 39, 169-177.

SCHWARTZ, M. *Stuttering Solved.* New York: McGraw-Hill Book Co., 1976.

SCHWARTZ, M. *Stutter No More.* New York: Simon & Schuster, 1991.

SCHWARTZ, M., AND CARTER, G. *Stop Stuttering.* New York: Harper and Row, 1986.

SCIENTIFIC AMERICAN. *The Brain.* New York: W. H. Freeman & Co., 1979.

SHAMES, G. H., AND FLORANCE, C. L. *Stutter-Free Speech: A Goal for Therapy.* Columbus, OH: Charles E. Merrill Publishing Co., 1980.

SHAMES, G. H., AND RUBIN, H., EDITORS. *Stuttering Then and Now.* Columbus, OH: Charles E. Merrill Publishing Co., 1986.

SHAPIRO, A. An electromyographic analysis of the fluent and dysfluent utterances of several types of stutterers. *Journal of Fluency Disorders,* 1980, 5, 203-231.

SHEARER, W. M. Speech: behavior of middle ear muscle during stuttering. *Science,* 1966, 152, 1280.

SHEARER, W. M. & SIMMONS, F. B. Middle ear activity during speech in normal speakers and stutterers. *Journal of Speech and Hearing Research,* 1965, 8, 203-207.

SHEEHAN, J. G. Theory and treatment of stuttering as an approach-avoidance conflict. *Stuttering Then and Now* (edited by Shames, G.H., & Rubin, H.). Columbus, OH: Charles E. Merrill Publishing Co., 1986, 187-200.

SMITH, A. Factors in the etiology of stuttering. *Research Needs in Stuttering: Roadblocks and Future Directions. ASHA Reports,* 1990, 18, 39-47.

SMITH, A. Neural drive to muscles in stuttering. *Journal of Speech and Hearing Research,* 1989, 32, 252-264.

SNYDER, M. A. The etiologies of stuttering. *Psychological & Psychiatric Aspects of Speech and Hearing.* Springfield, IL: Charles C. Thomas, 1960.

SODERBERG, G. The relations of stuttering to word length and word frequency. *Journal of Speech and Hearing Research,* 1966, 9, 584-589.

SPRINGER, S. & DEUTSCH, G. *Left Brain, Right Brain.* San Francisco: W. H. Freeman, 1981.

STARKWEATHER, C. W. Stuttering and laryngeal behavior: A review. *ASHA Monographs,* 1982, 21, 1-45.

STARKWEATHER, C. W. *Fluency and Stuttering.* Englewood Cliffs, N.J.: Prentice-Hall, 1987.

STARKWEATHER, C. W. Current trends in therapy for stuttering children and suggestions for future research. *Research Needs in Stuttering: Roadblocks and Future Directions. ASHA Reports,* 1990, 18, 39-47.

STARKWEATHER, C. W., FRANKLIN, S., & SMIGO, T. M. Vocal and finger reaction times in stutterers and nonstutterers: Differences and correlations. *Journal of Speech and Hearing Research,* 1984, 27, 193-196.

STARKWEATHER, C. W., & GIVENS-ACKERMAN, J. *Stuttering.* Austin, TX: Pro-Ed, 1997.

STARKWEATHER, C. W., HIRSCHMAN, P., & TANNENBAUM, R. S. Latency of vocalization: Stutterers v. nonstutterers. *Journal of Speech and Hearing Research,* 1976, 19, 481-492.

STRUB, R. L., & BLACK, F. W. *Organic Brain Syndromes: An Introduction to Neurobehavioral Disorders.* Philadelphia: F. A. Davis Co., 1981.

SUGARMAN, M. NSP going strong: a little history. *Letting Go,* July 1990, 3-4.

SUGARMAN, M. NSP going strong: a little history — Part II. *Letting Go,* Aug. 1990, 5-6.

THOMPSON, R. F. *The Brain: An Introduction to Neuroscience.* New York: W. H. Freeman & Co., 1985.

TORTORA, G. J., & ANAGNOSTAKOS. *Principles of Anatomy and Physiology.* New York: Harper & Row, 1981.

TRAVIS, L. E. The unspeakable feelings of people with special reference to stuttering. Emotional factors. *Stuttering Then and Now* (edited by Shames, G.H., & Rubin, H.). Columbus, OH: Charles E. Merrill Publishing Co., 1986, 93-122.

VAN RIPER, C. *The Treatment of Stuttering.* Englewood Cliffs, N.J.: Prentice-Hall, 1973.

VAN RIPER, C. *Speech Correction: Principles & Methods.* 6th ed. Englewood Cliffs, N.J.: Prentice-Hall, 1978.

VAN RIPER, C. *The Nature of Stuttering.* 2nd ed. Englewood Cliffs, N.J.: Prentice-Hall, 1982.

WEBSTER, R. L. Evolution of a target-based behavioral therapy for stuttering. Stuttering therapy from a technological point of view. *Stuttering Then and Now* (edited by Shames, G.H., & Rubin, H.). Columbus, OH: Charles E. Merrill Publishing Co., 1986, 397-414.

WEBSTER, R. L. *Fluency Master Procedures.* Hardy, VA: Epic Corp., 1989.

WEBSTER, R. L. *Precision Fluency Shaping (Vol. 1).* Roanoke, VA: Communications Development Corporation, 1974.

WEBSTER, R. L., & STOECKEL, C. M. *Precision Fluency Shaping Program: Speech Reconstruction for Stutterers.* Roanoke, VA: Communications Development Corporation, 1987.

WEBSTER, W. G. Hurried hands and tangled tongues. *Neuropsychology of Stuttering* (edited by Boberg, E.). Edmonton, Alberta: University of Alberta Press, 1993, 73-111.

WEBSTER, W. G., & POULOS, M. G. *Facilitating Fluency: Transfer Strategies for Adult Stuttering Treatment Programs.* Edmonton, AB: Institute for Stuttering Treatment & Research, 1997 (reprinted from 1989 work of same title originally published by Communication Skill Builders, Tucson, AZ).

WEINER, A. Vocal control therapy for stutterers: A trial program. *Journal of Fluency Disorders,* 1978, 3, 115-126.

WEISS, D. M. Fluency enhancing systems . . . for free! *Letting Go,* Feb. 1992, 12, 2, 4-5.

WESTBROOK, J. B. "Fluency-aids." *Letting Go,* Oct. 1992, 12, 10, pp. 1, 6-7.

WHITE, P. A., & COLLINS, S. R. C. Stereotype by inference: A possible explanation for the "stutterer" stereotype. *Journal of Speech and Hearing Research,* 1984, 27, 567-570.

WILLIAMS, J. D. 2,000 years of therapy. *Speak Easy Newsletter* (Paramus, NJ), Fall 1989, 9, 3, 4-5.

WILLIAMS, J. D. Use of the Edinburgh Masker. *Speaking Out* (Canada), May 1991, 8, 5, 7-9.

WINGATE, M. E. Sound and pattern in "artificial" fluency. *Journal of Speech and Hearing Research,* 1969, 12, 677-686.

WINGATE, M. E. Effect on stuttering of changes in audition. *Journal of Speech and Hearing Research,* 1970, 13, 861-873.

WINGATE, M. E. *Stuttering: Theory and Treatment.* New York: Irvington, 1976.

WINGATE, M. E. Speaking unassisted: comments on a paper by Andrews et al. *Journal of Speech and Hearing Disorders,* 1983, 48, 255-263.

WOLPE, J. Systematic desensitization based on relaxation. Behavior therapy of stuttering: deconditioning the emotional factor. Systematic desensitization. *Stuttering Then and Now* (edited by Shames, G.H., & Rubin, H.). Columbus, OH: Charles E. Merrill Publishing Co., 1986, 337-359.

WOODS, C. L., & WILLIAMS, D. E. Traits attributed to stuttering and normally fluent males. *Journal of Speech and Hearing Research,* 1976, 19, 267-278.

WU, J. C., MAGUIRE, G., RILEY, G., FALLON, J., LACASSE, L., CHIN, S., KLEIN, E., TANG, C., CADWELL, S., & LOTTENBERG, S. A positron emission tomography [18F] deoxyglucose study of developmental stuttering. *Neuroreport,* 1995, 6, 501-505.

WU, J. C., MAGUIRE, G., RILEY, G., LEE, A., KEATOR, D., TANG, C., FALLON, J., & NAJAFI, A. Increased dopamine activity associated with stuttering. *Neuroreport,* 1997, 8, 767-770.

WYKE, B. The neurology of stammering. *Journal of Psychosomatic Research,* 1971, 15, 423-432.

YAIRI, E., AMBROSE, N. G., & COX, N. J. Genetics of stuttering: a critical review. *Journal of Speech and Hearing Research,* 1996, 39, 771-84.

YEAKLE, M. K., & COOPER, E. B. Teacher perceptions of stuttering. *Journal of Fluency Disorders,* 1986,. 11, 345-359.

YEUDALL, L. T., MANZ, L., RIDENOUR, C., TANI, A., LIND, J., & FEDORA, O. Variability in the central nervous system of stutterers. *Neuropsychology of Stuttering* (edited by Boberg, E.). Edmonton, Alberta: University of Alberta Press, 1993, 129-163.

YOUNG, J. Z. *Programs of the Brain.* Oxford: Oxford University Press, 1978.

ZACKHEIM, C.T. Phonological priming in young children's picture naming: holistic versus incremental processing. (Presentation at Nat'l Stuttering Ass'n Conference, Nashville, TN, June 2003).

ZIMMERMANN, G. Articulatory behaviors associated with stuttering: a cinefluorographic analysis. *Journal of Speech and Hearing Research,* 1980a, 23, 108-121.

ZIMMERMANN, G. Stuttering: A disorder of movement. *Journal of Speech and Hearing Research,* 1980b, 23, 122-136.

ZIMMERMANN, G. N. & KNOTT, J. R. Slow potentials of the brain related to speech processing in normal speakers and stutterers. *EEG & Clinical Neurophysiology,* 1974, 37, 599-609.

ZIMMERMANN, G., SMITH, A, & HANLEY, J. Stuttering: In need of a unifying conceptual framework. *Journal of Speech and Hearing Research,* 1981, 24, 25-31.

Index

(Page numbers in italics refer to diagrams or tables.)

A

Abdominal cavity, 16, *17, 18, 24*
Abdominal muscles, *22, 26*
Accent, speaking with, 87
Acceptance of stuttering, 100-101, 102, 121-122
Acquired stuttering, 3, 56, 66
Adam's Apple, *15*
Adaptation effect, 67
Adronian speech exercise, 129-132, *131,* 134
    benefits, 129-130
    modified Adronian, 132, 134
    phonation, 130-1341 *131*
    problems in practicing, 131-132
    resonant speech, 132, 134
Adults' reaction to child's disfluency, 57-58
Air conduction, 85
Air pressure
    articulation, 21, 35-36, 58
    effect on strength and rigidity, 24
    plosives, 35-36, 58
    pressure-reducing techniques, 82, 126-127, 135-136
    relation to stuttering, 58
Airflow, 19
    passive, 18, 19
Airflow technique, 82, 95, 106
Airflow therapy, 106
Allen, Woody, 87
Alprazolam, 93
Americans with Disabilities Act of 1990, 145
Anafranil, 93
Anal fixation theory, 50
Anal muscles, 25

Anal sphincter, *26*
Anticipation of difficulty, 46-47
Approach-avoidance conflict, 52
Aristotle, 4
Articulation, 20-22
Artificial fluency, 78, 94
Artificial stuttering, 85
Arytenoid cartilages, 15, 20, *20*
Atkins, Joseph P., Jr., 31
Attitude therapy, 100-101
Attitudes about speech, 57, 119-122
Auditory feedback, 82, 83-86
    effect on Valsalva-Stuttering Cycle, 84
Avoidance behavior, 47
Avoidance reduction, 102, 116-117

B

Barton, Clara, 4
Behavior modification, 8
Bethanechol, 93
Bilateral speech, 68, 74
Block correction techniques, 103-104
Blocks, 2, 34-36
    anatomy of, 34-35
    on plosives, 35-36
    prolongation of consonants, 36
    repetitive, 36
    silent, 86
    Valsalva tuning, 34-36
Bone conduction, 85
Botulinum toxin injections to larynx, 92
    effect on Valsalva maneuver, 92

Brain (in general), 61-76, *62, 63, 68*
    anatomy, 61-64
    arcuate fasciculus, 62, *63*
    association areas, 62, *63*
    basil ganglia, 62, *62,* 69, 75
    brainstem, 62, *62*
    caudate, 68
    cerebellum, 62, *62*
    cerebral cortex, 62, *62*
    cerebrum, 62, *62*
    corpus callosum, 62, *62*
    fissures (sulci), 62
    frontal lobe, *63*
    gray matter, 61
    gyri, 62
    hemispheres, 62
    hypothalamus, 75
    left striatum, 68
    limbic system, 62-63, *62,* 75
    longitudinal fissure, 62
    midbrain, 70
    motor cortex, 63, *63,* 70
    occipital lobe, *63*
    parietal lobe, *63*
    parietal-temporal-occipital area, *63*
    perisylvian zone, 62
    prefrontal area, 70
    premotor area (cortex), 63, *63,* 70
    speech centers (*see also* Speech areas of brain), 62-63, *63*
    supplementary motor area (see also that heading), 63, *63,* 68, *68*
    temporal lobe, *63*
    thalamus, *62,* 63, 75
    Valsalva mechanism, 72-76

white matter, 61
Brain characteristics of stutterers
   acquired stuttering, 66
   diffuse brain injury, 67
   function, 67-68
   hemispheric dominance (laterality), 68
   lesions, 67
   neurological deficits (see also that heading), 7-8, 68-70
   patterns of brain activity, 67-68
   physical defects, 66-67
Breath chewing, 99-100
Breath control techniques, 94-95
Breathing, 16, 19
   chest breathing, 16
   costal breathing, 95
   diaphragmatic or abdominal breathing, 16, 126-127
   irregularities in stuttering, 45
Broadway Danny Rose, 87
Broca's area, 62, *63, 70*
Bryngelson, Bryng, 102

C

Canadian Association for People Who Stutter, 109, 111
Cancellation, 104, 136
Carroll, Lewis, 4, 69
Chest muscles, 24, *26*
Choral (unison) speaking, 81
Churchill, Sir Winston, 4, 69
Circumlocution, 44
Citalopram (Celexa), 93
Clomipramine, 93
Clonic spasms, 36
Clonic stuttering, 36
Co-articulation, 21-22, 80
Cognitive therapy, 100
Columbat, 94
Commercial stuttering schools, 95
Communication skills, 144
Consonants, 20-21
   fricative, 21
   liquid, 21
   nasal, 21
   plosive, 21
   semi-vowel, 21
   types of, 20-22
   voiced and unvoiced, 130, *130*

Continuous phonation, 39, 106, 129
Coordination and timing of movement, 69
Costal breathing, 95
Coup de glotte (glottal attack), 21
Cranial nerves, 62

D

Darwin, Charles, 4, 69
Delayed auditory feedback (DAF), 78, 83, 84-85, 94
Demands on child exceeding child's capacity, 57
Demosthenes, 93, 139
Desensitization, 7, 103
   systematic, 104
Developmental stuttering, 3, 56-57, 66
Devices, mechanical and electronic, 93-94
Diaphragm, 16, *17, 18,* 19, 24
Dieffenbach, Dr., 92
Diffuse brain injury, 67
Disability, 145
Discrimination, 144-145
Disfluency, 3, 57
Distraction, 87, 90
Dopamine, 68
Drug therapy, 92-93

E

Easy onset, 82
Edinburgh Masker, 83, 94
Educating the public, 143-144
Effort
   display of, 52-53, 58
   exertion of, 10-11
   little required for speech, 20, 22
   relation to Valsalva maneuver, 24
Effort closure, 23-24, *23,* 27, 32, 70, 73
Ego-defect neurosis theory, 50
Elocution lessons, 93
Emotional factors, 52, 57
Employment discrimination, 144-145
Enhanced vocal feedback, 85
Epiglottis, 14, *15, 16*

Esophagus, 14, *15*
Expectancy neurosis therapy, 99-100
Experience, effect of, 64
Expiration, 16, *18,* 19
   forced, 18, 19
Expiratory phonation, 73
Eye contact, 117

F

Faith healing, 91
False vocal cords, 15, *15, 16, 17,* 23, *23,* 24, 27
Famous persons who stuttered, 4, 69
Fiberoptic nasopharyngoscope, 31, 69
"Fight or flight" response, 75
Fillers, 44
Fluency Cycle, 115-117, *118*
Fluency enhancing conditions, 78-88
   effect on Valsalva-Stuttering Cycle, 79-79
Fluency Master, 85, 94, 106
Fluency shaping (*see also* Fluency training programs and Precision Fluency Shaping Program), 8, 39
Fluency training programs, 105-107
   shortcomings, 106
Force
   and air pressure, 58
   and difficulty in phonation, 39
   excessive, 11
Forceful closures of mouth and larynx, 34-36, 47
Frequency altered feedback (FAF), 86, 94
Freud, Sigmund, 7, 96, 97-98
Freund, Henry, 11
Froeschels, E., 99

G

Genetic factors, 59-60, 65-70
   heredity, 65-66
   traits crucial to stuttering, 69
   twin studies, 66
George VI, 4
Glottis, 15, *16*

H

Habit formation, 45
Haloperidol (Haldol), 92
Hard palate, 14, *15*
Harrison, John, 87, 122
Hearing and stuttering, 83
   hearing defect theories, 86-87
Hemispheres of brain, 62, 68, *68*
   dominant (left side), 62
   non-dominant (right side), 63
Hemispheric dominance (laterality), 68
   bilateral speech, 68, 74
   emotional interference theory, 74
   relation to Valsalva mechanism, 74
Heredity (*see* Genetic factors)
Hesitations, 2, 38, 43, 57
Hollins Communications Research Institute, 105
Hormones, 75
H-reflex, 74, 75
Hypnosis, 91

I

Inspiration, 16, *18*, 12
Inspiratory speech, 69, 73, 82
Intelligence, 69
Intercostal (chest) muscles
   external, 16
   internal, 18
International Stuttering Association, 109

J

Jacobson, Edmund, 104
Jendrassik's maneuver, 27
Jones, James Earl, 4, 87
Junk words, 44

K

Kingsley, Charles, 109
Kingsley Club, 109

L

Laterality (*see* Hemispheric dominance)
Lamb, Charles, 4, 69
Language skills, 57, 69
Laryngeal reflexes, 69-70, 73-74
Larynx, 14-15, *15, 16,* 23, *23, 24, 26,* 69-70, 73-74, 92
   injections with botulinum toxin, 92
Lastovka, M., 74, 75
Learned behavior, 7, 51
Legato speech, 39, 106, 132
Light contacts, 82, 116, 119, 136
Lips, 14, *15, 17*
Ludlow, Christy, 92
Lungs, 16, *17,* 24, *24*

M

Masking effect, 78, 83-84
Massed practice, 93
Maugham, W. Somerset, 4, 69
Mechanical devices, 93-94
Mechanoreceptors, 35
Medical and surgical treatments, 92
Mental reaction to stuttering, 47, 49, 137-138
Metronome effect (*see also* Rhythm), 78, 81, 94
Metronome, miniature electronic, 94
Moses, 4
Motor unit, 31
Mouth, 14, *15,* 26
Muscles
   contraction, 31
   fibers, 31, *32*

N

Nasal cavity, *15, 17*
National Council for Adult Stutterers, 109
National Council on Stuttering, 109, 111
National Stuttering Association (National Stuttering Project), 108-111
Negative stereotyping, 143-144
Nerve pathways, 62, 64
   alternative, 74-75
   development of, 64
   Valsalva mechanism, 74-75
Neurological deficits, 68-70
   subgroups of stutterers, 70
   weakness vs. interference, 72-73
Neurological factors, 7, 57, 65-76
Neurological views of stuttering, 7-8, 65-76
Neuromotor tuning, 31-32, 34
   larynx, 38
   prephonatory, 38
   Valsalva mechanism, 32-39
Neurons, 61-62, *62*
   "all or nothing" principle, 31
   axon, *32, 61*
   cell body, *32, 61*
   dendrites and spines, 61, *61*
   excitability, 31
   mechanoreceptors, 35
   motor, 31, *32*
   myelin sheath, 61, *61*
   sensory, 32
   synapse, 61
   synaptic cleft, 61
   synaptic terminal, 61, *61*
   threshold level, 31, 62
Neurotransmitters, 61, 75
Newton, Isaac, 4, 69
Non-auditory feedback, 84
Novel ways of speaking, 94

O

Objectivity regarding speech, 100, 117, 137-139
Occlusion effect, 85
Olanzapine, 92
Onset of stuttering, 4, 56-57
Operant conditioning, 105
Oral fixation theory, 50

P

Pacemaster, 94
Passive airflow technique (*see also* Airflow technique), 106
Pebbles in mouth, 93
Pennsylvania Hospital, 31
Persuasion, 91
Pharynx, 14
Phonation, 11, 15, 19-20, *23,* 37-38, 116, 128
   difficulty or delay, 11, 37-38, 47, 69
   effect on fluency, 39, 116
   inhibition of, 34, 37-39, 73
   neuromotor tuning, 38
   Valsalva tuning, 37-39
Phonation therapies, 106

Plus Club, 109
Positive anticipation of speech, 115, 120
Positron emission tomography (PET), 67
Precision Fluency Shaping Program, 105-106
    targets, 106
Preparatory set, 103
Prephonatory tuning, 38
Pressure-reducing techniques, 82
Priestley, Joseph, 4
Progression of stuttering, 57-58
Prolonged speech, 80, 135-136
    effect of DAF, 85
Proprioceptive feedback, 84
Prosody, 106
Psychoanalysis, 98
    free association, 98
    transference, 98
Psychological factors, 50-53
Psychological views of stuttering, 7, 50-53, 97-101
    criticism of, 98
    stigma created, 98
Psychology of stuttering, 50-53
Psychoneurotic disorder theory, 50
Psychotherapy, 7, 97-100
Puborectalis muscle, 25, *26*
    relaxation of, 125
Pull-out, 103
Punishment, 91

R

Rational emotive behavior therapy, 100
Reaction speed, 69
    inspiratory speech, 69, 73
    vocal delays, 11, 37-38, 69, 73
Recovery
    spontaneous, 4, 59
    variability, 59
Rectal muscles, *24*, 25
Rehabilitation Act of 1973, 145
Relapse, 8, 106-107
Relaxation, 95, 104-105
    electromyographic (EMG) biofeedback, 105
    progressive, 104
Repetitions, 2, 36, 57-58
    air pressure, 58

progression of, 57-58
Repressed anger theory, 99
Repressed needs theory, 99
Research, need for, 75-76, 142-143
Rhythm (*see also* Metronome effect), 81, 94
Rib cage, *17, 18*
Risperidone (Risperdal), 92
Role playing
    effect on fluency, 87
    visualization, 121

S

Schwa, 58
Schwartz, Martin F., 106
Secondary benefits of stuttering, 52-53
Self-help for stuttering, 108-111
    support groups, 109-111
    versus therapy, 108-109
Self-image, 52, 87
Self-talk, 120
Sexual differences
    in prevalence of stuttering 4, 59
    in Valsalva mechanism, 59
Shadowing, 81
Silent blocks, 86
Silent (lipped) speech, 11, 37
    effect on fluency, 37, 78
Simple disfluencies, 57
Singing, 11, 39, 78, 80
Slowed speech, 80, 116
    effect of DAF, 85
Smith, J. Stanley, 109
Soft palate, 14, *15, 17*, 20
Speak Easy, Inc. (Canada), 109, 111
Speak Easy International Foundation, Inc., 109, 111
Speaking exercises, 93
Speaking to oneself, 78, 79
Speech
    basics of, 19-22
    importance of, 2
    mechanism, 14-16, *17*
    sequence of movements, 22
Speech areas of brain (*see also* Brain), 62-64, *63, 68*
    arcuate fasciculus, 62, *63*
    association areas, 62, *63*

Broca's area, 62, *63*, 70
    perisylvian zone, 62
    supplemental speech area, 63
    Wernicke's area, 62, *63*
SpeechEasy, 85, 86, 94
Spinal cord, 62
Stammering, 3
Stapedius reflex, 86
Starkweather, C. W., 58
Starters, 3, 44
Struggle behaviors, 43-44
Stutterer's Declaration, *121*
Stuttering
    acquired (*see* Acquired stuttering)
    age of onset, 56-57
    behaviors, 3
    blocks, 2, 34-36
    circumstances of, 9-10
    clonic, 36
    controversies, 7
    covert stuttering, 3
    definition, 3
    developmental, 3, 56-57
    direct and indirect symptoms, 42-43
    genetic factors (see that heading)
    heredity (*see* Genetic factors)
    impact of, 4
    origins of, 56-60
    paradoxes, 6
    physical effort, 2-4, 10, 11
    prevalence, 3-4
    progression of, 57-58
    repetitions, 2, 36
    symptoms, 10-11
    therapy (see also that heading), 90-111
    tonic, 36
    variability, 6, 9-11
    varieties of, 42-45
Stuttering Foundation of America, 108, 111
Stuttering Hexagon, 122
Stuttering modification therapy, 101, 103-104
Substitution of words, 44
Suggestion, 91
    post-hypnotic, 91
Supplementary motor area, 63, *63*, 68, *68*, 74
Support groups, 109-111
Systematic desensitization, 104

T

Tactile feedback, 84
Teeth, *15*
Teeth ridge, *15*
Therapy (see also specific therapies), 90-110
   behavior-oriented therapies, 102-107
   controversies, 90
   effectiveness, 108
   effects on the Valsalva-Stuttering Cycle, 90, 91-95, 98-101, 102-107
   history, 90-95
   psychological approaches, 97-101
   versus self-help, 108-109
Thoracic (chest) cavity, 16, *18*
Thyro-arytenoid muscle, 27, 92
Thyroid cartilage, *15*
Timing irregularities, 44
Tongue, 14, *15*
   surgical mutilation, 92
Tonic stuttering, 36
Trachea (windpipe), *15*, 16, *17*
Triggering impulse or signal, 32, 34
Twelve-step programs, 111

U

Unison reading or speaking (*see also* Choral speaking), 78, 81
University of Iowa, 96, 97, 100, 102, 103
Urge to try hard, 47, 52-53
   resisting, 115, 121-122
Uvula, 14

V

Valsalva, Anton Maria, 24
Valsalva Control, 114-139
   abdominal breathing, 126
   Adronian speech exercise (see also that heading), 129-132, *131*, 134
   approaching speaking situations, 134
   attitude, 119-122
   daily exercise routine, 133-134
   exercises for Valsalva control, 123-127
   Fluency Cycle, 115-117, *118*
   handling blocks, 136
   key suggestions, 135
   learning from experience, 137-139
   maintenance, 134
   phonation exercises, 128-132
   pressure-reducing techniques, 126-127, 135-136
   principles, 114-118
   responding to fear and other emotions, 139-140
   steps for speaking, 135-136
   Valsalva relaxation, 115-116, 125-126
   vocalization exercises, 128-129
   voluntary Valsalva, 124-125
Valsalva Hypothesis, 32-33, 141-142
   blocks and forceful closures of mouth or larynx, 34-36
   interference with phonation, 37-39
   laryngeal reflexes, 73-74
   right brain involvement, 74
Valsalva maneuver, 24-27, *24*, 32, 123-124
   in exertion of effort, 24-25
   in forcing things out, 25
Valsalva mechanism, 11, 23-27, *26*, 32
   and brain, 72-76
   neuromotor tuning, 32-39
Valsalva perspective on stuttering, 141-142
Valsalva-Stuttering Cycle, 46-49, *48*, 78-79
   effect of fluency enhancing conditions, 78-88
Valsalva tuning, 33-39, 47
Van Riper, Charles, 98, 101, 103
Ventriloquism, 87
Vestibular folds (*see* False vocal cords)
Verapamil, 93
Vicious circle, 46
Virgil, 4
Visualization, 104, 121
Vocal control therapy, 39, 106
Vocal cords (folds), 15, *15, 16, 17*, 19-20, *23*, 24
Vocal delays, 11, 37-38, 47, 69
   inspiratory speech, 69
Vocal Feedback Device, 94, 106
Vocal folds (*see* Vocal cords)
Voiced sounds, 20
Voluntary controlled repetition (VCR), 102-103
Voluntary stuttering, 101, 102-103
Voluntary Valsalva, 103, 124-125
Vowels, 20
   mouth positions for, *21*

W

Weiss, Dan, 85
Wernicke's area, 62, *63*
Western Michigan University, 103
Wingate, Marcel, 81
Words
   as phonation and movement, 47, 74, 84, 122
   misconceived as things to be forced out, 47, 74, 76, 84, 122
Working hypothesis, 32

X

Xanax, 93

Z

Zyprexa (olanzapine), 92